Gambetta Method

Common Sense Guide to Functional Training for Athletic Performance

by Vern Gambetta

with selected contributions by
Gary Gray, Jimmy Radcliffe and Jason Soncrant

© 2002 Gambetta Sports Training Systems, Inc.
www.gambetta.com

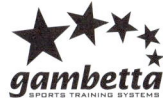

Library of Congress Control Number: 2002092930

ISBN: 1-879627-19-1

All rights reserved. Except for use in a review, the reproduction or utilization of the work
in any form or by any electronic, mechanical, or other means, now known or hereafter invented, including
xerography, photocopying, and recording, and in any information storage and retrieval system, is forbidden
without the written permission of the publisher.

The chapters in this book originally appeared as articles in *Training & Conditioning* magazine.
The articles in the compilation are the separately copyrighted property of MAG, Inc.

For more information, contact:
Gambetta Sports Training Systems, Inc., PO Box 50143, Sarasota, Florida 34232
Web site: www.gambetta.com

Cover: Photos by Dick Dickenson Studios, Vern Gambetta and Curt Gambetta
Book design and layout: Jennifer Ahearn-Koch, Sarasota, Florida

Introduction — Second Edition

The Gambetta Method is a compendium of articles that I have authored or co-authored for *Training and Conditioning Magazine* beginning in 1992. When I wrote the first article for the magazine, I had no idea that it would lead to a book. As I began to write more articles and receive feedback on the articles, a common theme began to emerge: the readers could apply the concepts because everything was very practical and functional. I took this for granted, because that is the way that I had always coached. We just called it training; now it is called functional training; which has become a commonly accepted approach to training and rehabilitating athletes.

The articles are in a sequence arranged by topic areas which reflect the progression through a systematic approach to training. Virtually every major aspect of training is covered, from planning to recovery to testing. Philosophically, this is not a rehash of conventional wisdom. Conventional wisdom is a starting point that should not limit our progress. The information represents a synergy of my interpretation of sport science research as well as my practical coaching experience. The concepts and ideas have been tested and proven on the courts, tracks and playing fields of the world. I am not saying that it is always correct, but in the words of Ralph Waldo Emerson: "Truth is what works." This collection also reflects the ability to ask the key question - Why? Without well-framed questions, we would never progress. It has been my experience that practice drives research. Practitioners cannot wait for research to tell them what to do; they must use the tools available and produce results. This book is about producing results!

During the course of my coaching career, I have had the opportunity to work or interact with some great coaches and sport scientists, as well as observe and train high level athletes in both individual and team sports. The common denominator among all of them was their desire to get better. Even though they were already the best at their respective jobs or sports, they were not satisfied with the status quo. They were constantly working to improve, to find a better way to get the job done. My wish is that this collection of articles will help you to improve so that you can be the best that you can be.

There are many people whom I want to thank for helping me throughout my career. All of the athletes with whom I have worked, from junior high school to world class, have taught me far more than I was able to teach them. Three stand out above the others—Kristen Engle, Lynne Hjelte, and Steve Odgers—because of what I learned from them and the way they approached sport and life. I have coached athletes with more natural ability, but few have come as close as these three to achieving their potential. Kristen has become a wonderful doctor, Lynn is a worldclass mother and wife and Steve is a great coach. I am thankful to have had the opportunity to work with all of them as well as with all the other athletes and coaches. I owe a special thanks to Red Estes, the former track coach at Fresno State, who encouraged me to go into coaching; Mr. Charles Kuehl, my high school basketball coach, who is still the best coach with whom I have ever worked, and Gary Gray PT, one of the most creative people I have ever known and a great human being who has helped me put it all together. Above all, I would like to thank my parents. They sacrificed so that I could get an education that they never had the opportunity to have. My only wish is that they could be here to read this. Their sacrifice and encouragement shaped me into what I am today.

I rededicate this book to my family, which has always given me unbelievable support: my wife, Melissa, who has stood by me all these years, always encouraging and supportive; and my children, Curt and Kristen, who make it all worthwhile.

Start by doing what's necessary, then do what's possible, and suddenly you are doing the impossible.
—St. Francis of Assisi

Forward — Second Edition

Steve Myrland, *Myrland Sports Training*,
Madison, Wisconsin

Vern Gambetta changed the way I do what I do. Of course, thousands can say the same; yet it is still important for me to acknowledge that this man has had the profoundest effect on how I work. This epiphany began in 1992 when I attended the inaugural *Building and Rebuilding the Athlete* seminar. I confess that I went into the experience with a poor attitude, expecting Mr. Gambetta to spend three days offering we attendees various strategies for enhancing the bench-pressing and power-cleaning abilities of the athletes we trained. I sat in the back row and listened. Vern got up and began to speak, progressively and methodically exploding the horizons I had been staring fixedly at for the first years of my coaching life.

He spoke about speed (in all directions), power, stamina, joint integrity, balance, agility, recovery, specificity, planning, and testing. He talked about the biomechanical requirements of different sports, athletic injuries (prevention and rehabilitation), and drew heavily from his extensive experiences and those of illustrious colleagues. When finished, he had given me more than new ideas to employ with my athletes: he had changed the way I approached my job. I was an excited young coach and I determined that this man would either have to tell me to get lost, or be willing to suffer fools gladly, for I planned to foist myself and my theories and questions on him at every opportunity thereafter.

Since some of what I now do involves speaking about performance and training, I have made it my business to attend clinics, seminars, and workshops with an eye to learning how to be a better presenter. I am persuaded that there are two main categories of teachers: the first are those who want you to *know* what they know; the second are those who want you to be *impressed* with what they know. Vern Gambetta falls squarely into the first category. His is a process of constantly questioning conventional wisdom, evaluating and re-evaluating the foundations of what he believes to be—if not the absolute truth—then the best truth available, and offering his conclusions—kindly—to anyone willing to listen. He makes his mistakes, learns from them; then helps the rest of us learn from them as well. You'll see: it's all here, in these pages.

When the history of training and human performance is written, rest assured that Vern Gambetta will be listed among the primary visionaries. I am grateful for his knowledge, his generosity in sharing it, and his patience in getting it to take root in the hard and unfertile ground that is, too often, my mind. And: I am unabashedly proud to call him my friend.

Steve Myrland-

Forward — First Edition

By Gary Gray, PT
Gary Gray & Associates Physical Therapy,
Adrian, Michigan

Vern Gambetta...friendship and function. These two simple words that have complex meanings come immediately to my mind. Vern is a friend in the true sense of the word, and his friendship is only superceded by his desire to become even more of a friend. Vern knows and has shared more about function than anyone I know. His functional wisdom is only superceded by his desire to learn and share even more about function. Within these pages you will learn about function. You will appreciate how much Vern knows about strengthening and conditioning and how he is able to apply his knowledge to enhancing the lives of others. You will realize the ability Vern has at sharing his wealth of information with us so that we can make a difference by helping others. More importantly, you will become aware of the wonderful caring attitude that defines Vern and is part of what makes him such a special friend. I am thankful that you have the opportunity to glean from Vern's wisdom and even more so thankful for Vern's friendship, dedication, and encouragement.

Table of Contents

A Tailored Program .... page 9
Following a Functional Path .... page 12
Fundamental Fun .... page 16
Athleticism — the Complete Athlete .... page 18
Get Ready, Get Set — Warm-up To Play .... page 21
Stretching the Truth .... page 23
Functional Flexibility .... page 26
Evolution Of Strength Training — a Personal Perspective .... page 29
Everything In Balance .... page 34
The Core Of the Matter .... page 36
Strength In Motion .... page 40
Strength By Design .... page 43
A Leg To Stand On — Training The Lower Extremity .... page 47
Prescription For Healthy Knees .... page 50
The Road To France — World Cup 1998 .... page 54
Round 'n' Round — Circuit Training .... page 58
More Power To You .... page 61
Leaps and Bounds — Progressing Into Plyometric Training ... page 64
Up, Up and Away — Vertical Jump Improvement .... page 69
Getting Gait Right .... page 73
In a Blur — Basic Speed Development .... page 76
Getting Up To Speed — Acceleration .... page 80
Multi-Directional Speed .... page 83
Sprint Drills — the Gerard Mach Way .... page 86
Speed Ways .... page 88
At the End Of Your Endurance .... page 91
Leading the Pack .... page 95
Rethinking Periodization .... page 99
A Plan Behind the Dream .... page 103
All Season Training .... page 106
Putting New Drills To the Test .... page 109
The Daily Special .... page 112
Team Training .... page 115
Breaking Through Plateaus .... page 117
The Perils Of Overtraining .... page 120
The Middle Years — High School .... page 123
Measure For Measure .... page 126
Evaluating Training .... page 130
Regeneration Gap .... page 133
Suggested Reading .... page 136

A Tailored Program

Getting your athletes in shape for their specific sports entails more than a progressive weight lifting and running program. To help athletes perform at their best, a conditioning program must be implemented that develops the athlete as a whole, while also taking into account his or her specific sport and physique. The following five-step program considers the sport, the athlete, the system, the plan, and the evaluation. It is a comprehensive system that can improve the performance of any athlete. The key is to take the general points explained here and turn them into a specific plan for your situation.

Step One: The Sport

Know and understand the sport for which you are conditioning. What is the metabolic demand? Is it primarily aerobic, anaerobic, or mixed? Is it weight bearing or non-weight bearing? What are the movement patterns? What muscles are used and how? What are the common injuries that occur and why? Is the work that you are using for conditioning specific and functional to the demands of your sport?

Planning a complete and competitive conditioning regimen for your athletes entails five major considerations....

It is surprising to me that more coaches do not take an in-depth look at their sport, or at the very least look at it differently. As Yogi Berra said, "You can see a lot by watching." Sometimes when I talk to coaches, I wonder if we are watching the same game. I urge you to take a close look from a different perspective, considering all the factors I have mentioned. You may find that the demands are different than you originally thought.

Generally, intermittent sprint and transition game sports require quick starts, rapid changes of direction, and quick stops. Aerobic endurance demands in most of these sports are minimal. For example, I analyzed a typical NBA game and determined that in the first half the ball was in play for an average of 49.1 seconds before action paused for an average of 35.3 seconds. In the second half, the average time of non-stop action was 37.5 seconds, with the average pause being 58.9 seconds. A top NBA power forward, one of the top rebounders in the league, only jumped 27 times during a game. Of those jumps, only a few were maximal jumps "above the rim!" Much of the running in the game is at a jog pace, and most of the players seldom run the entire length of the floor. Yet if one were to believe the hype and not carefully analyze the game, you would think of it as a continuous high-intensity game that is played "above the rim."

The same observations were made with other sports. In World Cup soccer play, even though the players averaged 10 kilometers run in a game, over 51 percent of the high intensity action lasted only 20 seconds or less. Actual sprinting during a match occurred only 5.8 percent of the time. In four-wall handball involving a world champion player, the mean game time was 17 minutes, with the ball in play an average of 47.3 percent of the time. The average length of each rally was nine seconds and the average pause was 10 seconds. Even though a championship tennis match may last four hours, the actual time of each point seldom exceeds five seconds in duration. Knowledge of facts such as these is essential to properly preparing athletes to compete in their chosen sport.

To analyze the patterns of movement of the sport, take a look at the joint sequence, large muscle usage, and alignment of the athlete's body during play. You can study the common injuries that occur in the sport by reading the injury records from past years. With all of this information in hand, you'll be able to set up a program that fulfills the needs of the particular sport.

Having knowledge of the sport is essential for properly preparing your athletes for competition. I urge you to take a close look at your sport from a different perspective. You may find that the demands are different than you thought. In the same vein, it may be necessary to analyze and debunk some of the commonly-used tests. In many cases, too much importance is attached to results that have little or no relationship to performance in the game. A 40-yard dash to measure football speed? A mile-and-a-half run to test endurance for a team sport? A 60-yard sprint to evaluate speed in baseball? A single maximum rep to test strength for sports other than weight lifting?

Beware of the myths about training and conditioning. Statements such as "the player has slow feet" or a "weak throwing arm" are commonly accepted. In actuality, the player probably has weak legs and a limited range of motion in the hips. The body is a link system and all parts work together from the toe nails to the finger nails. The feet or the arms do not operate independently of the rest of the body. So in the case of the above statements, improving leg strength and explosive power—as well as strengthening the core—will result in quicker feet and a stronger throwing arm.

You should condition for the "moment of truth." Even though the overall demand of the sport may be submaximal, the play that ultimately determines the outcome of the game will be decided by the player who can use his speed and quickness, despite the fatigue from the long match or game. Therefore, do not assume anything. Study and understand the movements, so that you will be better able to design a more functional program. A simple axiom is to train athletes, not workers. Condition with a purpose.

Step Two: The Athlete

Along with analyzing the sport, you'll need to study the specific athlete(s) with whom you work. How old is the athlete? How advanced is his or her skill level? What qualities does that athlete bring to the sport? What is their work capacity? What is their speed profile? What are his or her basic strength levels? What is their injury history? What about motivation? To answer these questions, talk to the athlete, look at his or her performance films, and review the athlete's testing information and injury history.

The difficult task for many coaches is having to accomplish this with a large number of athletes within the context of a team setting. The best solution to this problem is to use ability grouping: Group athletes on the team according to their abilities and have the different groups work on different skills and movements.

Ultimately, it is most effective to adapt the sport to the athlete rather than trying to adapt the athlete to the sport. The latter approach is doomed because it fails to take into account both the athlete's strengths and weaknesses. There is a tendency for coaches to concentrate on their athlete's weaknesses first. But, unless an individual weakness is so great that it does not allow the athlete to be effective and needs to be corrected, it is better to work on improving and emphasizing the athlete's strengths and minimizing the weaknesses.

Step Three: The System

The success of former Eastern Bloc countries in international competition over the years demonstrates the value of having a system for conditioning athletes. A system allows athletes with lesser natural ability to compete on an equal level with more gifted athletes because no aspect of preparation is ignored. A systematic approach implies a set order and procedure for training with all components taken into consideration. Without this, too much of the preparation is left to chance.

Your major task is to create a system of conditioning your athletes that works for the type of athletes that you have to work with and the facilities that you have available. Use your imagination and creativity to set up a program that is not limited by your facilities. What are your goals and objectives? Once you've determined the answer to this question, you can create an environment for conditioning where the athletes can only improve.

For optimum effectiveness, a training program must be multi-faceted. No component of training should receive emphasis over another until the athlete reaches an advanced state of development. When the athlete reaches that point, the emphasis should be on the area(s) that are hindering progress while at the same time stabilizing the strong areas. This is based on the principle of synergy, which dictates that the whole is greater than the sum of its parts. Therefore, no component of fitness will assume more importance than another in a well-balanced program. The key is balanced development between all components. The complete athlete is the product of a systematic training program that addresses all aspects of performance in order to achieve the highest level of athletic excellence.

A complete conditioning program will include all of the following components distributed throughout the training program in proportion to the athlete's needs:

Work Capacity — The ability to tolerate a high workload and recover sufficiently to perform the next workout or competition. This is sometimes considered synonymous with endurance. However, I believe it is more than that. It is related to the ability to perform for the required time with quality and efficiency, which is best developed for most sports through specific interval work and circuit training.

Speed — The ability to move the body or parts of the body as rapidly as possible without compromising the skill of the action. It can be summarized in one word: quickness. Aside from preparing someone to run a 100- or 200-meter sprint, the speed demands in team sports and individual sports like tennis and volleyball are brief three- to five-second bursts of activity with rapid changes of direction. It is best developed by performing quick bursts and allowing adequate rest between reps to ensure that the quality of performance is high.

Strength — The ability to exert force without regard to the time it takes to produce that force. Although this is an important area, it is over-emphasized in many sports. The principle means of developing strength is through weight training. It is important to establish a base level of strength.

Power — The ability to exert a great amount of force in the shortest possible time. I like to think of power as the ability to apply strength in the time frame required by the sport activity. The explosive effort required in most sports occurs in less than two-tenths of a second, which is well below the time necessary to develop maximum strength. Therefore, once a good strength base is achieved, the emphasis should be on functional activities like plyometrics and medicine ball training, which both raise explosive power.

Coordination and Skill Training — The ability to perform appropriate skilled action in proper sequence with perfect timing to produce a smooth flowing movement. This encompasses the area of fundamental movement skills and body awareness - an aspect often overlooked due to the necessity of working on specific sport skills. Fundamental movement skills can be easily incorporated daily as a part of warm-up in the form of drills that emphasize laterality, spatial awareness and joint proprioception.

There are numerous means of training to work each of the above components. Do not get carried away using a vast array of training methods. Each exercise should have a specific purpose in pursuit of a training objective. Stick with the basic "need-to-do exercises" in order to be most effective.

Step Four: The Plan

Decide on your specific training goals and objectives, then devise a plan and execute that plan. This process is called "Planned Performance Training". There is nothing mystical about this. It is simply detailed planning in pursuit of specific training objectives. Planning brings the future into the present so that you can do something about it. It helps to give a purpose and direction to the training and is basically something every great coach and athlete has done in their own way for years.

For some reason, the misconception has arisen that once the plan is written there should be no deviation, or the plan will not work. Nothing could be further from the truth. A plan must be flexible and adaptable to the changing needs of the athlete, otherwise, it is useless. Many people are intimidated by the jargon and terminology of planning, but the concept actually allows coaches to communicate in a common, consistent language.

The planning process is relatively simple in concept and application. Start by designing a macrocycle, which is a broad overview of the training year. Then, break that into smaller subdivisions called phases, which divide the year logically based on when the competitions occur. Usually there is a preparation phase, a competition phase, and a transition or active rest phase. The phases are broken into smaller periods called mesocycles. The mesocycle is usually three to four weeks in length. Mesocycles are broken down into shorter, more manageable periods of time called microcycles. The microcycle is usually a period of seven to 14 days. The microcycle is composed of training sessions made up of various training units. A training unit is work in pursuit of a specific capacity like strength, speed or power. The focus in planning should be on the microcycle and mesocycle, because those are the time periods that are most immediate and controllable for the athlete and coach. The yearly plan should be a broad overview, detailing the objectives for each phase, but not the specific workouts of the daily sequence.

Step Five: Evaluation

Evaluation should be an ongoing part of the training process. The evaluation must have a context, which is your plan. Evaluate the plan based on your objectives and revise as necessary. Decide what to test, how to test, when to test, and how to use the test results. Remember that testing is not an end in itself, but rather a means to the end of doing a better job of preparing the athlete for competition. Keep in mind that the ultimate test is performance in actual competition. Can the athlete perform at a higher level than he was able to achieve before the conditioning program?

The goal is to perform better. Best of luck! ◆

Following a Functional Path

Co-author: Gary Gray, PT

Are you doing leg curls for the hamstrings? Leg extensions and quad sets for the knee? William's flexion exercises and pelvic tilts for the back? Side lying external rotations for the rotator cuff? And have you asked yourself why you use these exercises?

It's true that there are the traditional exercises athletes have included in their regimens for years, but do they really work? The answer is a qualified "yes", but with very mixed results. If you perform these exercises over an extended period of time, the body will overcome the negative effects of the incorrect exercises. The key question to ask is: are the exercises functional?

Implementing functional training and rehab involves challenging conventional thought and focusing on the body's wisdom.

What is function? Function is what works! The term "functional training" is training that serves the purpose for which it was designed. In other words, it means training the respective muscle groups and involved areas to work in the same manner as they are used in activity. The term functional training has been around for a long time, but coaches are just now truly understanding its meaning and incorporating it into their training philosophies - with great results.

To truly understand function, it is necessary to cease focusing on artificial measurement and realize that the goal is to make the athlete better at his or her particular sport. Function involves the body's osseous system that provides structure, the muscular system that provides control, and the proprioceptive system that coordinates and directs movement. All of these are profoundly affected by gravity, ground reaction forces, and momentum. Where functional stability is concerned, isolated strength gains are minimized and the neuromuscular system is emphasized.

To implement functional training into a program, it is necessary to challenge conventional wisdom and understand the biomechanical aspects of function. It also demands imagination and creativity.

The best way to figure out the function of a muscle is to role play and become the involved muscle. Ask the muscle what it does in movement - not what it does in the anatomy book. For example, the conventional approach has been to train the extensor mechanism of the quads and patella to extend the knee. In function, however, the extension of the knee is performed by the soleus and posterior tibialis. When you talk to the patella and quadriceps as the foot hits the ground they will tell you what they do in function: they stabilize the knee and decelerate knee flexion. Follow this same thought process with other common movements and you will be surprised by what you find. The anatomy-book version of movement and the real-life version are very different.

Not surprisingly, functional training relates directly to the "Kinetic Chain" concept. The Kinetic Chain is characterized by deceleration at one joint and acceleration at the next joint in the chain. It also states that the muscles, joints, and proprioceptors all work synergistically — no joint or body part works in isolation. Therefore, it is important to train movements, not muscles. According to Johannes Noth in his chapter "Cortical and Peripheral Control," which appeared in the book *Strength and Power in Sport*, edited by Pavo Komi "the motor cortex is organized in such a way as to optimize the selection of muscle synergies and not for the selection of a single muscle. Thus...the motor cortex thinks in terms of movements and not muscles." Training individual muscles isolates and breaks the kinetic chain. Training movements integrates and improves the function of the kinetic chain.

In all motion, the body or a segment of the body will decelerate or reduce force before it accelerates to produce force resulting in the subsequent movement. In other words, performance is a constant interplay of force reduction and resulting force production occurring against a background of stabilization. In order for this to occur, the body takes advantage of gravity, ground reaction, and momentum. This concept is illustrated as the Performance Paradigm (See Figure One).

Implementing Functional Training
Functional training may be an unfamiliar concept to many coaches, but it does not require a radical change from current training programs. Rather, it requires looking at current training ideas in some new ways.

Sport Specificity — The purest form of training for any activity is the actual activity itself. Therefore, it is imperative that functional training include activities that are complementary to the sport being trained.

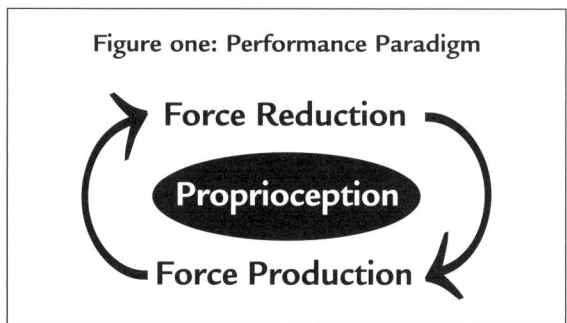

Figure one: Performance Paradigm

Performance Paradigm Descriptors		
Force Reduction	Proprioception Production	Force
Deceleration	Stabilization	Acceleration
Pronation	Joint Position	Supination
Eccentric	Joint Awareness	Concentric
Absorbing	Control	Propelling
Loading		Unloading

These should occur in multiple environments and include components of the actual function. The more functional the environments are in training, the more versatile the athlete will be in handling the forces and stresses incurred by the actual sport activity.

Proprioception — Functional training programs need to introduce controlled amounts of instability, which train the athletes to react to regain their stability. However, this training of the proprioceptive system should be as subconscious as possible so that the athlete is optimally stimulated by the imposed training demand. The task is to design activities that create an environment that is challenging enough to advance reactive function.

Gravity & Planes of Motion — The body's relationship to gravity must always be considered. Gravity is something that we cannot live without because it is constantly producing torque around all of the joints of the body. With respect to training, gravity's most fundamental and profound effect is on the body's posture. Standing and walking require that we overcome or, at the very least, neutralize the effects of gravity. Gravity is the basis of all resistance training. Therefore, we must learn to use it to our best advantage in all training situations.

With gravity also comes synergistic tri-plane motions at and between the various joints and synergistic tri-plane muscles functioning at and between the limb segments and the torso. Therefore, functional conditioning activities must also involve all three planes at all applicable joints at the same time. Specific planes of motion and specific joints can be emphasized with various activities, but all planes and joints must be integrated into the activities.

Loading — When considering loading and unloading activities for functional strength enhancement, always involve gravity as the primary form of resistance and then load the athlete intrinsically. This involves selecting activities so the body senses that the weight is coming from within or is part of the body. Once the body has adapted to this, add extrinsic loading to teach the body to react to forces from the outside. A practical example of this concept is to stress core before extremity strength and to use body weight for resistance before adding external resistance.

The initial load should be added eccentrically to teach the athlete to take advantage of force reduction in order to create force production. In addition, involve as many speed activities as possible. This will allow the athlete to take advantage of the eccentric load in order to produce a stronger and more powerful concentric action, resulting in more efficient movement.

Rehab — Movement can involve training an athlete to run, jump, or throw, or it can rehabilitate that same athlete from an injury. The principles of functional training apply to rehab in the same way they apply to conditioning. The body does not work any differently in rehabilitating from an injury than it did before the injury.

Open and Closed Chain — In function, there is no such thing as pure open and pure closed chain. All movement involves a coordinated opening and closing of the chain; the issue is not whether the movement is open or closed chain, but whether it is a functional or a non-functional movement.

Safety and Motivation — One of the most important principles of functional training and rehab is that the training must be safe and fun for the athlete. Safety can be guaranteed if the functional training program is based on the actual functionability of the athlete. And, as long as the athlete is working on functional patterns and movements that are closely related to the sport, the training will be fun and motivational because the goal will be intuitively realized on the part of the athlete.

Is It Functional?

The following are evaluative criteria to determine the extent that an activity may be functional:

Plane(s) of Movement — Does the motion involve tri-plane movement (Sagittal, Frontal, Transverse)? What plane dominates the movement and what phase of the movement does it dominate?

Joint Involvement — Single-joint movements that isolate a specific muscle are very non-functional. Multi-joint movements that integrate muscle groups into movement patterns are very functional. A very functional movement is when all joints are moving in all three planes simultaneously. If movement is limited at one joint, then movement must be focused at the joints above and below it.

Speed and Amplitude of Movement — The use of speed is often misunderstood in training and rehab. Traditionally the approach has been to start with slow, controlled movements. In functional training, the speed must be brought in slowly by controlling the movement. Speed is dangerous in training or rehab if it is focused on one joint. Speed is safe if its focus is multi-joint. For example, the 7,000-plus degrees/second torque at the shoulder in pitching is not produced at the shoulder, it is produced by the whole body and is expressed at the shoulder.

Proprioceptive Demand — This is the neural input from the joints, muscles, tendons, and other tissues that stimulate the functional movement patterns. It is the coordinator of the movement and the most important of all the criteria. The key to increasing function is to select exercises that have a high proprioceptive demand. It is possible to be strong, fast, or flexible, but if the proprioceptors are not developed to optimal level, movement will not be efficient, and the athlete will be predisposed to injury. In essence, it is proprioception that allows the whole to be greater than the sum of its parts.

Guided Resistance vs. Fast Eccentric Loading — Guided resistance such as that provided by most exercise machines places virtually no demand on synergists, minimizes the effect of gravity, and therefore has a low proprioceptive demand. Fast eccentric loading exercises, however, place a high demand on synergistic muscles and the proprioceptive system. In a controlled setting they teach the body to reduce greater forces more quickly to produce functional force patterns.

Progression

In functional training, progression is based on functional evaluation. Every activity is a test and every test is an activity. The training environment is the evaluative environment and the evaluative environment is the training environment. Similarly, the rehabilitative environment is the evaluative environment and the evaluative environment is the rehabilitative environment.

At the same time, however, it is important that the athlete is not constantly evaluating his or her own performance. Let the athlete perform and the coach, athletic trainer, or physical therapist evaluate. Movement must be spontaneous and subconscious. Imagine what would happen if a centipede started thinking which leg must move before the other.

The guidelines for progression in functional training involve emphasizing fundamental movement skills before the specific advanced skills. Overall, the progression in training and rehab should be:
- Basic Conditioning
- Basic Skill
- Advanced Conditioning
- Advanced Skill

When this progression is violated, at the very least, performance errors occur, and at the worst, injuries happen.

In addition, progression should not be based on an arbitrary or artificial timeline. Rather, it should be based on performance and objective feedback from the athlete performing the activity. Training and rehab is the process of devising strategies of getting the body to react.

In order to ensure proper progression it is helpful to apply the following criteria:

Simple To Complex — Start with simple exercises first and add complexity as the athlete adapts to and masters the movement.

Easy To Hard — Start with easy exercises and methods and increase the complexity as mastery of the easy movement is achieved.

Correct Execution To Increased Repetition To Increased Intensity — Do not allow the athlete to learn the movement incorrectly. Stress correct execution with an individualized cue system to help remind the athlete of correct mechanics.

Appropriate Functional Goals — Rather than a predetermined progression of sets and reps, the objective should be a series of functional goals that the athlete can use to measure progress toward the ultimate goal. Part of the goal is to see functional failure when compensations are occurring. Continue the activity until abnormal compensation begins to occur.

Injuries

The goal of training and rehab is to make the athlete better at his or her chosen sport or activity, but it is precisely the activity that causes improvement that can also cause an injury. Should an injury occur, how can we make the "causative activity" contribute positively to the athlete's development or rehabilitation? Essentially, we must realize that the causative activity is really what will make the athlete better in training and will be the cure if there is an injury. In both scenarios, the body must successfully deal with the loads and motions that are produced. The effective management of the apparent dichotomy is based on a sound fundamental understanding of the biomechanics of movement and the function of the entire kinetic chain.

The body instinctively has a weak-link focus. The cliché that the chain is only as strong as its weakest link can be applied to the concept of body movement. The body either breaks down at the weak link or transfers the force elsewhere in the body. When that force is transferred elsewhere, that body part is ready for the increased forces or has a breakdown. In a game, when one player gets tired, the coach will substitute another fresh player. The body works in a similar manner. This can be good or bad depending on the quality of the substitute and the demand placed on that substitute.

Methodology

Traditionally, the selection and use of methodology has been the focus in rehab and conditioning. In functional training, it is more important to understand the performance paradigm and the conceptual basis of functional training — and then be able to apply these ideas to your situation. It is also important to consider a spectrum of training or rehab activities that challenge the system to improve. Motion, stability, speed, flexibility, and strength are all facilitated concurrently; they are not developed separately and then combined. The body will adapt very rapidly with this type of training. Therefore, it is important to have a variety of activities that constantly force adaptation within the constraints of safety and common sense.

The choices of specific methodology are vast. Some easily accessible functional methods include free weights, medicine balls, tubing or stretch cords, manual resistance, and neurological stimulation. They are all viable methods if used within the context of the principles previously discussed. Remember that the methods are just the tools; without a plan and a trained user, the tools can be virtually useless.

To be most effective all methodology must meet the criteria of the "Three P's": 1) Is it Practical? Can it be accomplished given the level of development of the athlete and the facilities and equipment available? 2) Is it Personal? Does it meet the needs of the individual athlete both in terms of level of sport proficiency and physical development? 3) Is it Proactive? Is there a plan? Does it anticipate the possible roadblocks to progress and provide a method to overcome those obstacles? ◆

References:

Gray, Gary. *Chain Reaction Plus*, Wynne Marketing, Adrian, Mich., 1994.

Noth, Johannes. "Cortical and Peripheral Control" in *Strength and Power in Sport*, Pavo Komi, Editor, Blackwell Scientific Publications, London, 1992.

Fundamental Fun

For the past two generations of athletes, we have pushed early specialization in sport as the key to success. By the time of adolescence, if an athlete has not decided to focus on one particular sport, the thinking goes that he or she has little hope of ever making it to an elite or professional level.

Although it is difficult to assess the exact impact of this approach, I am beginning to see that it does have one major drawback: it occurs at the expense of learning fundamental movement skills. By age 12, many youth baseball players know how to throw a curve and lay down a bunt, but few can nab a line drive hit in an awkward spot. Similarly, young basketball players can make some amazing jump shots, but often play defense with very little grace or body awareness. When the athlete is asked to go outside the sport's narrow performance spectrum and extend to an unusual position or make an unfamiliar move, he or she often cannot.

Along with inhibiting athleticism, neglecting the teaching of fundamental movement skills may also be a leading cause of injuries. When the athlete is not correctly performing basic movements like running and throwing, overuse injuries and muscle pulls tend to occur. And when the athlete is not able to successfully complete an unfamiliar movement in the heat of competition, the result can easily be a twisted ankle or knee, or a collision-type injury.

One consequence of this may be the large number of ACL injuries in female basketball and soccer players. The lack of preparation is not in basketball or soccer skills, but in general conditioning and fundamental movement skills. Another example is the number of elbow and shoulder injuries in young baseball players. Watching the Little League World Series this summer, I saw a group of youngsters who were proficient at baseball but deficient in movement skills. They were good players for their age, but their running ability and throwing mechanics were noticeably weak. It left me questioning how much better they can get without developing better movement skills and if they will be able to stay injury free.

For me then, it comes down to this: are we asking athletes to play games they are not prepared to play? They seem ready in sport movements, but they often come up short in the prerequisite fundamental skills. Success is built on fundamentals, and the most basic fundamental of all is movement skill.

Reintroducing Fundamentals

Addressing this problem will require rethinking athletics for children, both in school curricula and the emphasis on competitive youth teams. It also applies to how we currently coach our high school, college, and elite athletes.

In the past, movement skills were often learned through free play and reinforced in physical education classes. However, in our society today, free play has almost disappeared. When was the last time you saw a group of children playing tag in a field? Today's children are more sedentary, and when they do play, it is in an organized game or practice session for their sport. They are often driven in cars to practice, where they used to walk or ride bicycles. It is not surprising to watch the Olympics and see African distance runners dominate or athletes from Brazil and Nigeria excel in soccer — movement is more a part of their lifestyle than in our culture.

The solutions require us to begin making changes at the lower-school levels. The ideal scenario would be to reinstitute mandatory physical education from K-12 in every state. In these classes, a range of movement abilities could be fostered through play and self-discovery as the child grows and develops. A national run, jump, and throw program could also teach and reward the mastery of these basic skills.

In the short term, youth-sport coaches must incorporate fundamental movement skills as a routine portion of their practices. There are optimal sensitive periods for the development of different elements of fundamental movements of which coaches need to be aware. For example, balance is best developed at ages 10 to 11 for boys and ages 9 to 12 for girls. Fundamental movement skills developed at these younger ages become automatic and part of a reservoir of motor skills that can be called upon when learning specific sport skills. So when should specific sport skills be introduced? It really depends on the sport, as some sport skills can be introduced earlier than others. The key is to look at the sport skill and analyze it in the context of what movement skills must first be mastered in order to perform it. Then design a progression so that there is a smooth transition from one into the other.

One overall rule for any such progression is that speed must be incorporated first. Because it is a motor quality that demands a high degree of coordination, speed must be mastered before almost any skill movements are added. It can be developed in a play environment using tag games and relays, keeping everything short and quick so that fatigue is not a factor.

It is important to remember that these fundamental skills are not just for children, though. Coaches at every level should be teaching and reinforcing these movements daily. Practicing proficiency in movement should not be regarded as a step backwards in the learning curve, but rather as a basis for more complex sports skills and as a means of injury prevention and performance enhancement.

Breaking It Down

What are the basic fundamental movement skills? They consist of the following broad categories:

Locomotor Skills are skills that move the body from one place to another. They consist of walking, running, leaping, hopping, and jumping.

Nonlocomotor Skills involve little or no movement of the base of support. Also called stability skills, they consist of movements like swaying, turning, twisting, swinging, and balancing.

Manipulative Skills are movements that focus on control of objects primarily using the hands and feet. They are both propulsive and receptive. Propulsive skills include striking, throwing, and kicking. Receptive skills include catching and trapping.

Movement Awareness includes those abilities needed to conceptualize and form an effective response to sensory information.

Body Awareness is the knowledge of one's own body parts and their movement capabilities. It includes the following components:

Spatial Awareness is the understanding of how much space the body occupies and the ability to orient to other people and objects in space.

Rhythmic Awareness is the ability to make movements that are repetitive and patterned, resulting in balanced, harmonious movement.

Directional Awareness is the ability to discriminate the size of objects and their relation to each other. Directional awareness also includes what I like to call "laterality" (awareness of right and left) and directionality (awareness of forward-back and up-and-down and other various combinations).

Vestibular Awareness provides information about the body's relationship to gravity. It is the basis for balance and body position.

Visual Awareness is the ability to receive and process visual stimuli.

Temporal Awareness is the timing mechanism in the body.

Auditory Awareness is the ability to discriminate, associate, and interpret sound.

Tactile Awareness is the ability to discriminate through touch and feel.

At all levels, these movement skills should be incorporated into all facets of the workout. Various fundamental movements can be practiced during a structured warm-up, with the practice session slowly leading up to more sport-specific movements. The optimum order of development is to first learn the movement without any regard to speed. Next, increase the speed of the movement while paying particular attention to maintaining the precision of the movement. The third step is to change the movements or do them under slightly different conditions. The fourth step is to follow with fundamental sports skills based on the movement skill.

In a youth-sports situation, the focus should be primarily on the first three steps. In teaching soccer, as an example, practice sessions should center around locomotor skills: all sorts of running, leaping, and jumping games should be performed using the ball more as a prop than as a variable. For example, have the athletes run 10 yards, jump over the soccer ball, then run another 10 yards. They can then perform the same drill at a faster pace. In the third drill, scatter soccer balls in various patterns on the field and have the children run over to them as fast as they can while maintaining balance. They can also play chasing games, attempt to balance in fun ways, and enjoy moving their feet in new patterns.

At more advanced levels, soccer practice can begin with the players running cone drills and conducting lateral movements at a controlled pace. The athletes can then hasten the pace, still focusing on balance and control. Next, the drills can be altered slightly or made more random—visual or auditory response can also be added. Finally, the athletes can try performing the drills while dribbling a ball or they can use the learned movements against a defender.

The above ideas may seem to be a step backwards—fundamentals are what we did 20 years ago, and "sport-specific" is the current concept. However, fundamentals should really never have been allowed to slip out of our programs. In our haste to have our athletes achieve success in their sports, I think we have ended up neglecting these basic movement skills. It's time to bring them back. ◆

References

Drabik, Jo'zef, PhD, *Children and Sports Training*, Stadion Publishing Company, Inc. Island Pond, Vt. 1996.

Gabbard, Carl, Leblanc, Elizabeth, and Lowy, Susan, *Physical Education for Children — Building the Foundation*. Prentice-Hall, Inc. Englewood Cliffs, N.J. 1987.

Athleticism — The Complete Athlete

Where have all the athletes gone? At first, that may seem like a very naive — or wildly exaggerated — statement, but let's examine it further. We have basketball players who can slam dunk but cannot execute a basic pivot move; quarterbacks who can throw a seventy-yard pass but can't avoid an onrushing lineman; baseball players who can hit forty-plus home runs in a single season but who cannot play defense. How have we gotten to this state? What is missing? In a word, athleticism. We know it when we see it. We all talk about it. But what is it? Why is it declining? And, how do we reverse this decline and develop athleticism in our athletes?

Let's begin by defining the term. Given its widespread use in the world of sports performance, I was surprised that I was unable to find an acceptable definition. So I came up with the following: Athleticism is the ability to execute a series of movements at optimum speed with precision, style, and grace.

It is certainly not a complicated definition. It is easy to see when someone has athleticism. But throughout the world of sport, even though performance standards continue to skyrocket, we are seeing less and less athleticism. Why? There are several factors that have led to the decline in athleticism. Here are the main ones, with some suggestions of what can be done to correct them.

Causes and Remedies

Early specialization in one sport and even in one position or event within a sport is a serious problem that has contributed to this decline. This is the downside of the emphasis on specificity in training as well as the emphasis on early specialization. Sometimes we are led to believe it is an either/or proposition. Produce a better athlete, or produce a better sport player with refined specific skills. But, ultimately, athletes must have both — the goal is to produce the best possible athlete who plays a particular sport. In this way, not only will performance be enhanced, but injuries will be reduced.

Some people argue that there is an apparent conflict in terms of time and effort: one school of thought feels that with the same amount of training time available, it's just not possible to train to improve athleticism without sacrificing specific-skill training. We need to eliminate the distinction — the two are not mutually exclusive. They are co-dependent and intertwined — one enhances the other. Training must have a purpose. Mainly, the training must transfer to the game. With a base of athleticism, specific training will be even more purposeful.

Many people have forgotten about the importance of the broader range of motor skills developed through free play and exposure to many varied motor programs. There should be time within the context of the existing structure of any training program to fit in components of athleticism. It just needs to be made a priority.

The New York Times sports pages of Sunday, November 12, 2000, had a great article on the University of Connecticut women's basketball that highlighted the value of athleticism. There was a section on Kelly Schumacher, the starting center, who attended a small school in Quebec where she participated in a number of sports. "Unlike athletes from larger cities who often are forced to specialize early," the article stated, "Schumacher played a number of sports at tiny Pontiac High School in the town of Shawville, where she was part of a graduating class of 50. Soccer helped her footwork and agility. Volleyball refined her timing for blocking shots in basketball. She won a tennis tournament in her first attempt, her mother recalled, and she made an intimidating opponent in badminton. She even learned to play the fiddle, and step dancing honed her keen sense of balance." No doubt, all of these experiences helped make her one of today's top college women's basketball players.

One-sided training with an emphasis on one or two components of performance rather than a blend. The components of performance, and therefore training, are speed, strength, stamina, suppleness, skill, and recovery. There is a synergistic relationship among all components. Therefore, all components must be trained during all phases of the year in varying combinations.

The Highlight-Play Syndrome has led to an erosion of fundamentals. The young athlete is trying to be spectacular rather than fundamentally sound. But games are made up of hundreds of average plays that are more important than the one highlight that gets on television. Focusing on good, sound athletic development will prepare the athlete to make the average play consistently and the spectacular play when needed.

"Monkey See — Monkey Do" Syndrome. Just because an athlete or a team has been successful with a particular training method does not mean that the method is the best or that it should be copied. It is my experience that many athletes and teams are successful in spite of — not because of — their training. Make sure that what you are doing is based on sound training principles and a good progression.

Nobody gets hurt, but nobody gets better. Training that

> *While many athletes impress with a few flash moves, the best are those who can do it all. Here are the pitfalls to avoid and the best ways to develop an all-around athlete.*

is so conservative or narrow that the athlete is never challenged will not produce results. The justification for many machine-oriented strength-training programs is that they are "safe." In fact, they might actually predispose the athlete to injury because they fail to challenge his or her athleticism.

Further, the fact that we live, work, and play in a gravitationally enriched environment cannot be denied. Over-reliance on machines will give us a false sense of security because they negate some of the effects of gravity. Gravity and its effects must be a prime consideration when designing and implementing a functional training program; otherwise, we are not preparing the body for the forces that it must overcome. We cannot ignore gravity; it is essential for movement.

Therefore, we must learn to overcome its effects, cheat it, and even defeat it occasionally.

A Return To Athleticism

It is always easy and convenient to look to the "good old days" as being better. But, sometimes, it really is worthwhile to look back to gain perspective and insight into how to move ahead. The simple fact is that before the advent of specialization, athletes at the high school level, and even at the college level, participated in several sports. It was not unusual to see a high school athlete play football, basketball, and baseball, or run track. The athlete may not have been as good in any one sport early on, but once he or she did choose to specialize, he or she had a broader base of motor skills to draw upon to enhance specific sport skill. We cannot go backward,

Fitting In Athleticism

Where do you put athleticism training in a team workout? Start with the first step of the workout. You need to warm up every day before every training session. Make the warm-up the start of your daily dose of athleticism training. An extensive, well-planned, dynamic warm-up can set the tempo for that day's practice. This should consist of a variety of running patterns, skips of all different varieties, side-stepping, and backward runs. These all should be done in a progressive manner with one movement flowing into the other. Have your-athletes warm up in this way every day and you'll soon see a positive training effect.

It is best to develop various modules that address each of the fundamental movements that are the precursors for sport skill. I suggest that you have two to three modules that you can utilize both in warm-up and that are then also spaced at strategic intervals throughout practice.

Let's take balance as an example. The following balance modules were developed by Steve Myrland of Myrland Sports Training in Madison, Wisconsin:
Basic Balance (do these drills on firm, flat ground):
Static balance (standing still) on each foot.
Progress to barefoot, repeat with eyes closed, then add an unstable surface such as a foam pad.

Dynamic Balance: Forward step to balance on each foot. Backward step to balance on each foot. Lateral step to balance on each foot. Transverse step (turn and step) to balance on each foot. Repeat with eyes closed, then add an unstable surface such as a foam pad.

Ballistic Balance: Forward bound to balance on each foot. Lateral bound to balance on each foot. Backward bound to balance on each foot. Transverse (turn and bound) to balance on each foot.

Balance Circuit Stepping Stones: Place a group of small medicine balls unevenly spaced about two to four feet apart. The athlete must step from one to the other without touching the ground.

Footwork: The footwork component of agility can be addressed daily through use of the agility ladder. The following are three footwork modules that can be used as part of a warmup or incorporated as breaks throughout practice:

Agility Ladder Footwork Module I
Forward 2 In
Forward 1 In
Lateral 2 In
In/In - Out

Agility Ladder Footwork Module II
Two ladders three-to-five meters apart — any combination of drills. Pick four to five drills (repeat each drill twice)

Jump Rope: Another great daily athleticism activity is jumping rope. It develops hand/eye and hand/foot coordination and combines the elements of balance and footwork. It is also more beneficial than jogging to raise core temperature. Use a variety of patterns of jumps. Follow that with two to three sets of multi-direction jumps. These consist of a jump forward immediately followed by a jump sideways, followed by a jump sideways in the opposite direction, followed by a jump back.

but we must look for ways to enhance athleticism that has been lost due to early specialization.

The basis of training athleticism is rooted in running, jumping, and throwing — three actions that encompass the whole spectrum of human movement. It is imperative to look for every opportunity to incorporate these elements in all aspects of training. This doesn't mean a whole new set of training exercises and drills. Keep in mind the saying, "You don't need to see different things, but rather to see things differently."

Athleticism can be developed through a systematic approach to athlete development. Specific sport skills are a combination of patterns of complex motor programs. They are patterns that can be reproduced when we tap into the wisdom of the body. Through experiencing all different patterns of movement we learn to let things happen. We learn to let the motor program run efficiently. We learn how best to cue an action that will result in a "chain reaction" of efficient movement. In order to develop this fluidity and improvisational skills, we need to emphasize a free-play approach.

The body is a link system, often referred to as the kinetic chain. Athleticism training is all about linkage — all the parts of the chain working together in harmony to produce smooth, efficient patterns of movement. The brain does not recognize individual muscles. It recognizes patterns of movement, which consist of the individual muscles working in harmony to produce movement.

Should we try to teach every movement and then coach it? Or, should we allow the athlete the joy of discovery through exploration? There seems to be a concern about athletes getting it wrong. But, what is wrong? In all athletic endeavors, there must be a spontaneity and anticipation, not a robotic, programmed approach. It has been my experience working with athletes at all levels in a wide variety of sports that athletes will find their own best way of doing something if they are put in a position where they have to adapt. We need to encourage an extemporaneous approach that will allow each athlete to develop his or her way to solve the problems presented in sport activities — much like a great jazz musician improvises.

Understanding and training athleticism is a challenging process. It demands creativity and imagination. It is often contrary to conventional wisdom as represented in current mainstream sport science research that emphasizes specificity and measurable outcomes. Do not be limited. Use conventional wisdom as a starting point and move forward while thinking and acting outside the box. You and your athletes will more greatly enjoy the day-to-day challenges of training — ultimately resulting in a higher, more injury-free level of performance. ◆

> *We need to encourage an extemporaneous approach that will allow each athlete to develop his or her way to solve the problems presented in sport activities — much like a great jazz musician improvises.*

Get Ready, Get Set — Warm-up To Play

As they walk onto the field or court before a game or practice, athletes tend to do one of two things: they either pick up a ball and start throwing, shooting, or kicking without any preparation to play, or they plant themselves down on the ground and proceed to stretch for 20 minutes. Athletes call this their warm-up. However, neither approach is a successful way to warm up the body. There is an alternative to both of these traditional warm-up routines. This alternative requires a methodical approach, in which you examine the workout/competition slated for that day and then structure the warm-up to match. This allows proper preparation for training and competition and thus can be a key element in the athlete's ultimate success or failure.

Why Warm Up?
The warm-up may be the most important component of the whole workout because it is a bridge between normal daily activity and training. A good warm-up will prepare the athlete for a sound workout, as well as set the tempo for the workout. A poor warm-up will result in a sub-par workout or, at the very least, will cause the first part of the actual training to be performed at a less-than-optimum level. What happens is that the body attempts to warm up during the training. A 15 to 20-minute warm-up daily is a significant accumulation of training time over the course of a training year.

One final reason not to short-change the warm-up: when put in the context of total training time for the year, warming up will occupy one-fourth to one-fifth of the training time.

Consider all the things a proper warm-up can do:
- Help to prevent injury.
- Raise core temperature of the body.
- Raise the level of excitation of the nervous system.
- Improve elasticity and the contractile ability of the muscles.
- Improve efficiency of the cardio-vascular and respiratory systems.
- Shorten reaction time.
- Enhance overall coordination.
- Regulate the emotional and arousal state.
- Raise work capacity.

Because the warm-up is so important, it must be as thoroughly planned as the workout itself. It must allow a seamless flow into the actual training session, and it must dovetail with the planned objective of the training session. Therefore, it is important to vary the warm-up based upon the objective of the actual workout. The mindset must be that the workout starts with the warm-up; it is not a separate part.

Most athletes equate warming up with stretching. the truth is, a proper warm-up entails much, much more.

Also note that when working with young athletes, a good thorough warm-up can comprise the entire workout. The first few training sessions should consist of little more than an extensive warm-up with an emphasis on correct execution of the exercises and a routine of preparation to play or train.

One more point before we get into the specifics: stretching is not a warm-up! Stretching may be part of a thorough warm-up, but only if it is active and dynamic, as opposed to static. According to Thomas Kurz, in *Science of Sports Training* (Stadion Publishing Co., 1991), "Doing static stretches before a workout that consists of dynamic actions is counterproductive. The goal of the warm-up, which is to improve coordination, elasticity, and contractability of muscles and breathing efficiency, cannot be achieved by doing static stretches, isometric or relaxed. Isometric tensions will only make you tired and decrease your coordination. Passive, relaxed stretches, on the other hand, have a calming effect and can even make you sleepy."

Components of a Warm-up
A proper warm-up can consist of a wide variety of exercises. The key is choosing those that will enhance the workout to come. In determining your warm-up routine, consider the components listed below, thinking about the content of the actual workout, the location of the workout within the weekly training cycle, and the needs of the individual athlete.

Light Aerobic Activity — This involves three to five minutes of continuous rhythmic activity, which can be light running, jumping rope, StairMaster, or bike riding. The goal is to raise the core temperature of the body.

Loosening — Use large-amplitude movements incorporating flexion/extension, rotation, and bending. These movements are dynamic, not ballistic. The emphasis should be on rhythm, gradually working to the end range of movements. Exercises should include leg swings, arm circles, and trunk rotations. The goal is to lubricate the joints.

Balance — This component should incorporate both static and dynamic balance activities. Use a combination of balance beams, foam rollers, and balance single-leg squats. The goal is to heighten proprioception.

Flexibility — This involves range of motion with control. Stretches should be held for one to two seconds. The emphasis should be on the muscle groups that undergo the most stress. It is not necessary to stretch every muscle of the body, as that would be an inefficient use of warm-up time. The goal is to improve range of motion.

Coordination — Always work on fundamental

movement skill before specific sport skill. Emphasize rhythm and tempo of the exercise. These should be total-body movements of large amplitude. The goal is to address fundamental movement skills to improve body awareness and coordination.

Core Work — Incorporate flexion/extension, rotation, and diagonal rotational patterns with this component. This can be done with body weight, medicine balls, weight plates, stretch cords, or body blades. These warm-up exercises are especially important preceding a strength-training session. The goal is to improve awareness and control of the center of the body.

Specific Warm-up — For this one, simply incorporate sport-specific movements at a lower intensity. The goal is specific preparation for the actual workout.

Cooldown — This is a mirror of the warm-up and helps the athlete transition back to normal daily activities. The goal is to accelerate recovery and restore the body back to its pre-workout state in order to prepare for the next training session. Always think of it as a cooldown, not a shutdown.

How Much Time?

The length of the warm-up can range from 15 to 40 minutes, depending on the main emphasis of the workout and the training task that immediately follows the warm-up. For speed, strength, and other workouts that have high technical demands, the warm-up should be long. Warm-up for endurance sessions or workouts of low technical demand can be relatively short. Also consider environmental conditions in the length of the warm-up. A colder day will require more warming up than a hot day.

The second and third warm-ups of the day, if multiple training sessions are planned, do not have to be as long as the first, provided they are not separated by more than six to eight hours. The body remains metabolically active, so each succeeding warm-up after the first can be reduced in length.

Pre-Competition Warm-up
The pre-competition warm-up has some similarities to the pre-practice warm-up, but needs to be longer and even more thorough. Less time is devoted to general warm-up and more time is devoted to specific warm-up. In the early season, plan longer warm-ups, and as the season progresses the warm-up time can be reduced and the content changed to reflect the changing demands of competition. As a general rule, begin the warm-up 60 to 70 minutes before the start of the actual competition.

The pre-competition warm-up can play an important role in controlling competition anxiety and arousal. If the athlete is overanxious and nervous, then the warm-up should include more stretching and calming activities. If the athlete needs to be more "psyched up," then the warm-up should be more vigorous and active.

Before competition be sure to allow enough time for all particulars, including a period for individual time if it is a team warm-up. Don't forget to factor in athletes' personal needs, such as changing into dry clothing, using the rest room, or putting hair in a braid. Carefully plan back from the start of the competition so that all elements have sufficient time.

The following are sample warm-ups:
Basic Warm-up
Skip 2 x 30 yds
Sidestep 2 x 30 yds
Long & Low Carioca 2 x 30 yds
Carioca 2 x 30 yds
High-Knee Carioca 2 x 30 yds
Backward Run 2 x 30 yds
Straight-Leg Prances 2 x 30 yds

LSA Warm-up
High Skip 2 x 30 yds Lateral Speed & Agility Warm-up
Serpentine Run 2 x 30 yds
Diagonal Plant & Cut 2 x 30 yds
360s 2 x 30 yds
Touches (alternate hands) 2 x 30 yds
Sprint/Backpedal 2 x 30 yds
Backpedal/Sprint 2 x 30 yds Dynamic
  Change-of-Direction Warm-up
Skipping: use a reaching arm action (one arm
  & two arm), then a crossing arm action
Crossover Skip
Crazy Hips
Sidestep: switch direction every two;
  also perform at angles
Carioca: switch direction every two;
  also perform at angles
Leg Swing Out & Around Hip Mobility

Advanced Warm-up
Karate Squat
Carioca Skip
Side Skip
Side Walking Lunge
Giant Step: forward & back, to the side, crossover
Forward/Back Out & Around
Hurdle Walks: hurdle walkovers and out
  & around walkovers
Diagonal Kicks: bent knee, then straight leg
Crossover Bound: straight leg then bent knee
Zig Zag Bound Continuous Warm-up: Combine all
  components of previous warm-ups and continue
  for a target time. Usually 10, 15, or 20 minutes.
  Use this warm-up on a day when the workout is
  lower intensity. ◆

Stretching the Truth

Perhaps the most misunderstood and controversial component of training is flexibility. Much of this controversy has arisen because of the myth that flexibility is a panacea—that our athletes must become contortionists in order to prevent injuries and perform athletic movements. This is a gross misrepresentation of the role that flexibility plays.

To be sure, flexibility is an important piece of the training puzzle, but like other aspects of training, it must be based on the sport and the individual. Being able to stretch body parts into pretzel-like positions is great for a gymnast, but may be counterproductive for the soccer player.

Before we ask our athletes to prove their elasticity in a sit-and-reach test, we must ask ourselves the following questions: Where is flexibility needed and how is it most efficiently developed? How much of flexibility is determined by joint structure and body structure? What is the best time in the workout to develop flexibility? What are the flexibility requirements for various sports? Is it possible to be too flexible?

Static vs. Dynamic

The conventional definition of flexibility is the range of motion that is available at a particular joint while the body is at rest. For most athletes, however, such a definition is not particularly relevant. During competition, the athlete's body is not at rest — and this can change a joint's range of motion.

Instead, flexibility during movement must be viewed as a dynamic controlling quality: it allows the joint to go through as large a range of motion as can be controlled. The controlling nature of flexibility governs two areas: the range of motion used in skill performance and the length of the movement available for force production and reduction.

To conceptualize this idea, I use the term "mostability," which is a synergistic combination of motion and stability. Gray defines mostability as "the ability to functionally take advantage of just the right amount of motion at just the right joint in just the right plane in just the right direction at just the right time" (Gray, 1996). The opposite is instability, which is any degree of mobility that cannot be controlled.

Perhaps the reason flexibility is thought of as a static quality is that it is often measured statically by factors such as the sit-and-reach test. However, experience as well as research has shown that there is no relationship between static flexibility and dynamic performance. Some of the fastest and most explosive athletes that I have worked with have been "tight." Conversely, some of the most-often injured athletes were the individuals who were most "flexible" in the conventional sense.

In addition, the dynamic range of movement expressed in sports movements is significantly greater than can be expressed statically. This is due to the elasticity of the involved tissue and reciprocal inhibition, which allows the opposing muscle group to relax. Such is why a pitcher can externally rotate at the shoulder beyond 90 degrees when pitching, but statically may not be able to get within 10 to 15 degrees of that dynamic range.

Functional Flexibility

So what is the goal of flexibility training? Essentially, it is to functionally increase and strengthen range of motion. Therefore, the athlete's sport must be considered and his or her joint strength must be an integral component of flexibility training.

Flexibility is a dynamic not a static quality. Therefore it must be improved dynamically.

Consider the following quote on flexibility and sport-specificity: "...While there is no proven connection between joint looseness and overall athletic performance, too much looseness can be a real liability in sports that require rapid changes of direction and acceleration, such as basketball, tennis, and soccer, while too little of it would seriously restrict a gymnast or a figure skater; and so the quality of joint looseness or flexibility is largely sports specific" (Arnot and Gaines, 1984).

After sport-specific considerations, we must understand the relationship between flexibility and strength. According to Kreighbaum and Barthels: "Flexibility ... is an important factor in prevention of injuries and in efficient skill performance, but to satisfy these purposes, flexibility must be accompanied by ligamentous and muscular stability surrounding an articulation .... Adequate strength in extreme joint positions also is necessary to prevent joint structure damage by the outside force" (Kreighbaum and Barthels, 1990).

Observing these concepts will give the control and range of motion necessary to efficiently and safely perform the required skill. Most importantly, joint integrity must never be compromised for range of motion. When this occurs the athlete will be predisposed to injury.

Also important to note is that improper strength training can impair flexibility. This is not because the athlete becomes too muscular or muscle bound, although that is a possibility, but because the improper development of a muscle or a group of muscles around a joint can result in a restriction of motion at that joint. My personal experience is that a properly designed strength-training program will enhance flexibility rather than retard it because of the control and stability that strength lends to movement.

Assessing the Athlete

Assessing the athlete is the first step in flexibility training. To begin, one must understand the factors that influence an athlete's flexibility. Flexibility is both an anatomical quality and a physical ability. Anatomically, it is determined by the shape of the joints. Physically, it is the ability to perform movements through a large amplitude.

Furthermore, consider the following five factors that determine flexibility:
- The elasticity and the length of the involved muscles and tendons. This is determined genetically but can be altered through a well-designed strength-training program.
- The structure of the joints. The shoulder is inherently more flexible than the knee or hip because of the structure of the articulation.
- The level of basic coordination allowing motor control of the involved joints.
- The fitness level of the athlete.
- The psychological/emotional state of the athlete. The athlete who is 'uptight' or tense by nature tends to be less flexible.

Formally assessing flexibility is best done through the observation of athletes in their respective sports. Functional flexibility is best exhibited by economy of movement in the desired sport skill — the athlete who is too tight will not have this economy of movement. Ask yourself: Is the athlete smooth in his or her movements? Can he or she get in the required positions dynamically? Has there been a pattern of injuries?

If the answers to these questions point to a deficiency, then it is time to do a more detailed functional assessment. The tests should be functional and dynamic and must make comparisons intra-individual rather than inter-individual. For example, compare left to right to identify any deficiencies. Observe the athlete's movements and see if deficiencies identified on the tests impair performance in any way. The results are highly individual, therefore we should not compare flexibility norms.
What about the traditional sit-and-reach test? Fundamentally, it is a mistake to include the sit-and-reach on the President's Physical Fitness Test battery (for the previously mentioned reasons). What makes it even more fallacious is to have norms set that make inter-individual comparisons on this highly individual physical quality.

What are better ways to test flexibility? Consider the tests in the book *Lower Extremity Functional Profile,* by Gary Gray with Team Reaction, as a beginning point to developing your own functional flexibility profile. I do not think we should try to come up with a universal flexibility test that addresses all populations. It is more useful and practical to develop a test that measures "mostability" in positions that the athlete will have to perform in competition.

Developing Flexibility

When gains in flexibility are needed, they should be developed individually for each athlete. Here are some principles to follow:

- Use moderation and common sense. Flexibility is only one component of fitness—do not overemphasize it.
- Do not force a stretch. If it hurts, don't do it.
- Flexibility and strength training should be combined.
- Be joint-specific in the development of flexibility.
- Emphasize dynamic flexibility.
- Do not use bouncing ballistic stretches.
- Orient the body in the most functional position relative to the joint or muscle to be stretched and relative to the athlete's activity.
- Use gravity, body weight, and ground-reaction forces as well as changes in planes and proprioceptive demand to enhance flexibility.
- Develop a flexibility routine specific to the demands of the sport and the qualities of the individual athlete.

Unlike other physical qualities, flexibility can be improved from day to day. And once range of motion is increased or developed to the desired level, it is easy to maintain that range of motion. Less work is needed to maintain flexibility than is needed to develop flexibility.

When?

Many of the problems with flexibility begin with its placement within the structure of the workout. Too many coaches equate stretching with warming up. However, stretching is not warming up. You must warm up in order to effectively stretch and gain flexibility.

Out of habit, many athletes perform static stretching during their warm-up. But static stretches before warm-up or competition can actually cause tiredness and decrease coordination. In addition, static stretching improves static flexibility, while dynamic stretching improves dynamic flexibility. Therefore, it is not logical to use static stretches to warm up for dynamic action.
The optimum time to develop flexibility is post-workout. Muscles are already warmed up; consequently the greatest gains can be made at this time. Post-workout flexibility training also has a regenerative effect, calming the athlete, restoring the muscles to their resting length, stimulating blood flow, and reducing spasm.

In *Stretching Scientifically — A Guide to Flexibility Training,* Kurz presents a convincing argument for including an early morning stretching session in a flexibility program. This session simply entails performing a few rhythmic dynamic stretches to lubricate the joints and should take 10 to 15 minutes. Kurz recommends that no isometric static stretches be done in the morning because they are too exhausting to the nervous system. "The purpose of this stretching is to reset the nervous regulation of the length of your muscles for the rest of the day" (Kurz, 1994). The athletes that I have used it with have felt that it helped them better prepare for workouts later in the day.

Age Development
The work of Drabik highlights the growth and development considerations for flexibility. At preschool age there is no need for any development as natural play and movement take toddlers' joints through full ranges of movement. From age six through ten, the mobility of the shoulder and hip is reduced. Therefore, to prevent any permanent reduction in mobility at these joints it is necessary to do dynamic stretches. Drabik recommends: "[avoid] static stretches of all kinds (passive, active, isometric) in training preadolescent children because excitation dominates over inhibition in a child's nervous system. This means that it is hard for children to stay still, relax, and concentrate properly on feedback from their muscles for periods as long as static stretches require" (Drabik, 1996).

Age 10 to 14 is the developmental stage where flexibility should receive emphasis. With the rapid growth that occurs in this age range, flexibility should focus on the muscles made tight by the rapid growth of bones. If this is not done, the ultimate effect will be bad posture and susceptibility to injury. After the growth spurt, flexibility training can be increased and become more sport-specific, very similar to an adult program.

Conclusion
There have certainly been some great athletes who have also been able to exhibit amazing flexibility. However, this is not usually why they are great athletes. Athleticism combines strength with coordination, of which flexibility can be useful in certain situations. The goal of flexibility training is not a "Gumby" effect where the athlete has no joint integrity, but rather strength intertwined with flexibility that allows the athlete to control his or her movements. Performance is not a stretching contest! ◆

References:
Arnot, Robert B., and Gaines, Charles L., *SportsTalent*, Penguin Books, New York, N.Y., 1984.

Dominguez, Richard H., and Gajda, Robert S., *Total Body Training*, Warner Books, New York, N.Y., 1982.

Drabik, Jo'zef, *Children and Sports Training*, Stadion Publishing Company, Inc., Island Pond, Vt., 1996.

Hartmann, Jurgen, and Tunneman, Harold, *Fitness and Strength Training*, Berlin, Sportverlag, 1989.

Kreighbaum, Ellen, and Barthels, Katherine M., *Biomechanics — A Qualitative Approach for Studying Human Movement*, Third edition, Macmillan Publishing Company, New York, N.Y., 1990.

Kurz, Thomas, *Stretching Scientifically — A Guide to Flexibility Training*, Stadion Publishing Company, Inc., Island Pond, Vt., 1994.

Kurz, Thomas, *Science for Sports Training — How to Plan and Control Training for Peak Performance*, Stadion Publishing Company, Inc., Island Pond, Vt., 1991.

Functional Flexibility

By Jason Soncrant, PT and Vern Gambetta

Flexibility often conjures images of slow meditative movements, deep breathing, and muscles stretched taut like rubber bands. In describing flexibility, words and pictures are commonly used that convey a static position or still picture.

This is precisely where many misconceptions about flexibility begin. Flexibility for sports is more than maximal lengthening of soft tissue — and it is not a posed, static position. It is about movement and control of multiple positions that must occur rapidly to meet the demands of an athlete's sport. It is a very important component of sport performance that can be significantly improved if approached correctly.

Sport-specific flexibility requires an integrated expression of joint stability, strength, movement awareness, and soft tissue extensibility. What good is soft tissue flexibility without joint stability? What good are supple muscles if they cannot control segmental body weight as the athlete fights gravity? What good is any of this if the body cannot interpret external sensory input to promptly initiate a coordinated sequence of segmental movements? The muscles must be flexible, but they must also be able to initiate and control the athletic actions sports demand.

The flexibility program is based on the most fundamental movement, the gait cycle. This is the basis for all movement, from walking to running to jumping, and even throwing. The phases of the cycle describe movement as it passes through weight acceptance and limb advancement in both single or double-leg support. Each phase of the gait cycle puts different demands on the muscles crossing the various joints that produce movement and joint stabilization. The stretches that we describe are designed to address those demands. They have direct application to all sport activities. The first thing to understand is that,

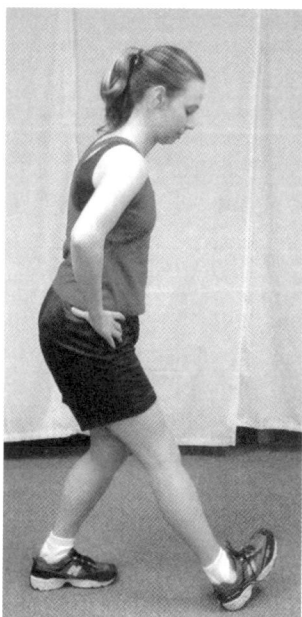

Figure One: Hamstring stretch for initial contact

These stretches performed in sequence help to prepare the body for locomotion by addressing multi-joint and triplanar balance and flexibility.

in gait, all joints are moving simultaneously and in all three cardinal planes. Therefore, stretching to improve gait requires multi-segmental and triplanar movements against gravity with neural excitation. Also, realize that the stretches are not static. Stretches must include joint movement even when the muscle is lengthened, because that is how they function in gait. Muscles are stretched to provide eccentric segmental stabilization long enough for forward momentum and concentric muscle action to create segmental mobility elsewhere in the body.

Below, each basic phase of gait is listed with a brief description followed by practical stretches that apply to the muscles used in that phase.

Initial Contact

This is the starting point, where the reference foot contacts the ground, starting a double-leg support phase. Typically, the heel strikes first and ahead of the pelvis. The impact causes the ankle to plantarflex with knee and hip flexion. There is rapid internal rotation of the femur and tibia relative to the pelvis. The hamstring and hip rotators act to decelerate these sagittal and transverse plane movements.

Stretch — Perform a typical standing hamstring stretch with internal and external hip rotation of the limb being stretched. We call this a bottom-up stretch because it is being driven from the ground up. Start in the standing position, place one foot a comfortable step-length in front of the other, either on the ground or on a six-inch step. The knee and hip are slightly flexed with the ankle maximally dorsiflexed. The stance leg is held in a relatively straight position. In this position, you may feel pulling in the back of the thigh or calf. While maintaining this posture, rotate the leg being stretched in and out. If done correctly, you will feel the intensity and location of the stretch change with the rotation. Hold the stretch for 10 seconds. (See Figure One)

Loading Response

Continuing in double-leg support, the pelvis moves forward and downward toward the lead foot. The lead foot is flat on the ground, which allows the ankle to dorsiflex while the hip and knee continue to flex and internally rotate. The hamstrings, posterior calf, quads, and hip rotators are all active in controlling these movements.

Stretch — Standing, place one foot on a six-inch step. The front knee is flexed roughly 50 to 60 degrees, with the ankle dorsiflexed. The rear leg should be straight, with toes pointed slightly inward. Reach across your body until you feel a stretch into your lumbar, gluteal, and hamstring regions. Your opposite elbow should come in close proximity to your reference knee. The lead arm should not reach to the floor, but should reach horizontal to the floor. Hold the stretch for 10 seconds. This is a top-down stretch because the arms drive it from above. (See Figure Two)

Midstance

The body assumes a single-leg stance as the pelvis moves directly over the reference foot. The opposite foot is off the ground and swings forward past the reference foot. The ankle is relatively dorsiflexed and abducted, but the calcaneus is starting to invert, the knee is extended with the hip extending, adducting, and internally rotating. The unsupported side of the pelvis rotates forward past the supporting limb.

Stretch — Start in a single-leg stance standing tall. With your foot flat, drive your pelvis forward. Your belly button should now move over your toes, thereby lengthening the posterior calf and anterior hip soft tissues. Don't excessively arch the back. Now, step forward with the opposite leg 12 to 20 inches ahead of the supporting foot. Allow only the heel of the front foot to contact the ground to keep the bodyweight on the back leg. The stretch should be felt in the gluteal and lateral hip area of the stance leg. Hold for five seconds in each position. This is a balance stretch. Allow your pelvis to glide forward over the fully planted foot to mimic continued forward momentum of the pelvis. (See Figure Three)

Terminal Stance

The opposite foot is on the ground in front of the reference foot, creating a double-leg support phase again. The reference hip trails behind the opposite hip. The reference hip must extend, abduct, and internally rotate to allow forward momentum of the freely swinging limb to continue. While the reference ankle is inverting, it is moving from a dorsiflexed and abducted position into a plantarflexed and adducted one.

Stretch — Assume a stride position, with one foot in front of the other in a straight line. The length of the stride should be about the same as leg length. Be sure to keep the back heel down and the front knee bent. To stretch the psoas, gently rotate your shoulder to the right and then repeat to the left. To stretch the calf, toe in on the back foot 30 degrees. Now, drive your hips forward so that most of your bodyweight is on the lead foot. Repeat the stretch with the rear foot toed out 30 degrees. Hold each position for 10 seconds and repeat five times. (See Figure Four)

Pre-swing

Remaining in double-leg stance, the reference foot is pulled off the ground by forward momentum of the pelvis. Normally, the heel lifts first and then the toes. The moment the toes clear the ground, this phase ends. The hip is still extended, abducted, and externally rotated. The knee flexes to help clear the foot. The ankle plantarflexes, abducts, and inverts. The toes, especially the hallux, must go through a large excursion.

Stretch — Assume a lunge position with the back foot on a four- to six-inch step. Be sure your feet are oriented in a straight line. Now, in a controlled fashion, glide your hips forward to pull the rear heel off the step. Allow the heel to rise until most of the pressure is on the toes and balls of the feet. Be sure to keep the toes planted so they bend sharply. (See Figure Five)

Swing Phase

Concentric muscle activity drives this part of gait. The entire time, the reference limb swings forward through the air until the moment before the foot contacts the ground, usually with the heel, thus ending one cycle and immediately flowing into the next cycle. The reference side of the pelvis is unsupported and rotates forward with the swing limb. Forward locomotion is strongly propelled by the swing-limb momentum.

Stretch — The leg swings while in single-leg stance. Allow the swinging leg to angle about 30 degrees across midline while pointing the toes straight ahead. The key to this stretch is to, at the same time, exaggerate arm swing to accentuate core rotation in swing phase. (Figure Six)

Conclusion

These stretches performed in sequence help to prepare the body for locomotion by addressing multi-joint and triplanar balance and flexibility, in single- and double-leg support. Both open and closed chain events are targeted and the eccentric and concentric muscle activities are addressed. If any of these factors

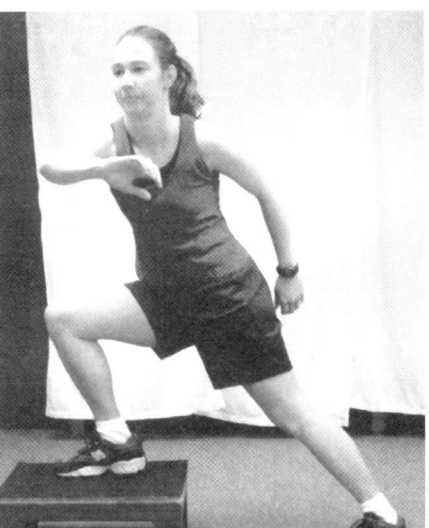

Figure Two: Stretching out the lumbar, gluteal, and hamstring regions for the loading response phase

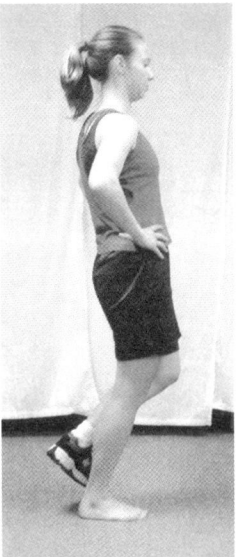

Figure Three: A midstance stretch

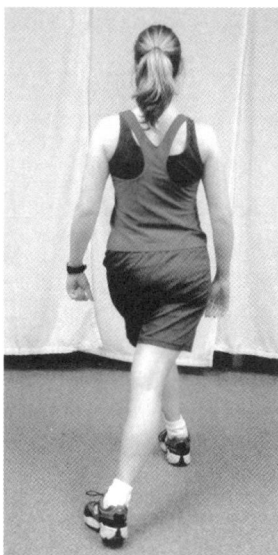

Figure Four: Stretching the calf for the terminal stance phase.

are missing or reduced, then the overall gait efficiency is impaired. If one phase of gait is removed, the body has to create drastic and inefficient strategies to compensate.

For example, to limit the loading response, try walking slowly and perform initial contact with the entire foot. You will feel slow and awkward. Your step length is shortened and you probably will increase your arm swing and hike your hips to compensate. Now try walking fast. The relative extension in the joints reduces effective shock absorption and you may feel more impact into your back and the strain in your hips.

Next, try eliminating the terminal stance and pre-swing phases of gait. Walk in a goose-step fashion by swinging your legs in a limited fashion. The arc of swing is from just under your hips to in front of them. Walk slowly, then fast. You will not feel very swift and you are likely to bound upwards in order to generate forward momentum. You can feel your abdominals and hips straining. Your hamstrings may also feel a little snug. This gait alteration has caused you to fail to pre-stretch the abdominal and anterior hip/thigh muscles to create

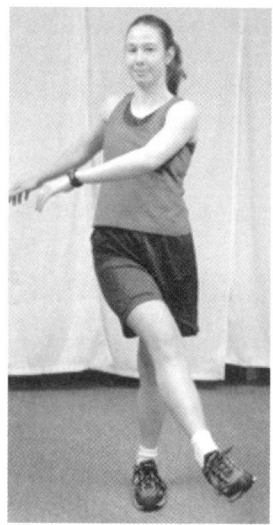

Figure Six: : Leg and arm swings to stretch the core in the swing phase

an efficient and powerful swing phase.

The amazing thing about gait is how each phase of the cycle translates so smoothly into the next phase. Success at one phase of gait is heavily influenced by the previous phase.

Because the gait cycle is the basis for all movement and its components play such an active role in sport performance, basing flexibility training on gait maximizes results. With these few simple stretches, athletes will be able to achieve maximum flexibility with the most crossover to actual sport movements. ◆

Further Reading

Norkin, C., Levangie, P. *Joint Structure & Function: A Comprehensive Analysis.* 2nd Ed. F.A. Davis: Philadelphia, 1992.

Tiberio, D., Gray, G.W. "Kinematics and Kinetics During Gait." In Donatelli, R., Wood, M.J., eds. *Orthopaedic Physical Therapy.* Churchill Livingstone: New York, 1989.

Root, M.L., Orien, W.P., Weed J.H. *Normal and Abnormal Function of the Foot.* Vol II. Clinical Biomechanical Corp.: Los Angeles, 1977.

Gray, G.W. *Chain Reaction Festival Seminar.* Wynn Marketing, Inc.: Adrian, MI. 1996.

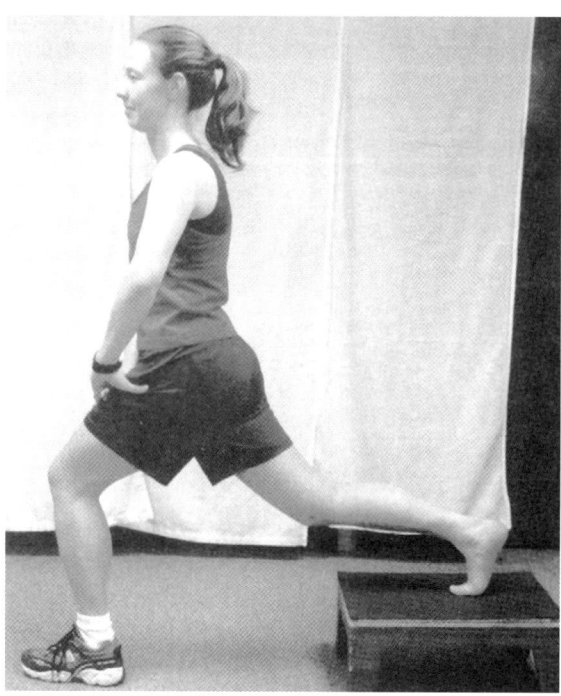

Figure Five: A stretch for the preswing phase

Evolution Of Strength Training — a Personal Perspective

When I began weight training in 1963, it was not commonly accepted as a method of training — in fact weight training was discouraged. There were concerns that you would become "muscle bound," that it would slow you down, or it would interfere with your coordination. It was considered acceptable to do hard manual labor to develop muscle, but weight training was frowned upon. With all these thoughts in mind, we had a guest speaker come to my high school to speak to all the athletes. The speaker was Lynn Hoyem, a backup center for the Dallas Cowboys, who spoke to us about the benefits of weight training. He had gained 50 pounds of lean mass through weight training. He gave us advice on how to start a program and explained some of the basic physiology of muscle growth and strength gain. He offered tips on how to gain weight, as most of us were football players who were trying to do so. It was a very impressive presentation that was very different from what we were being told at the time. I knew that if I were going to have any chance of playing college football, my sport of choice at the time, I would have to get stronger and bigger.

At that time, there was not very much information on weight training. Before I started on a strength training program, I felt I needed to find out more information because my coaches were very wary of weight training. My best friend and I went to the local university library and checked out every book they had on weight training. The two books that I found most helpful were *Weight Training In Athletics and Physical Education* by Gene Hooks, who was the baseball coach at Wake Forest University and *Better Athletes Through Weight Training* by Bob Hoffman, who was the owner of York Barbell company and a pioneer in weight training. The books were very good and gave us the information we needed as to selection of exercises, sets, reps, and overall construction of a weight training program as well as reinforcing that weight training would help us be better athletes. In addition, *Strength and Health* magazine, published by Bob Hoffman, proved to be a good source because it contained high level information on all aspects of strength training, including tips on good nutrition. The information was very good. In fact, it was cutting edge with the latest training ideas from the eastern bloc countries and features on top athletes who made use of weight training in their training programs. It was very informative and motivational because they were working hard to break down the myths surrounding weight training.

After gathering as much information as I could, building some basic equipment and purchasing a barbell set, my best friend and I started on a program. When I began I weighed about 163 pounds. I was so tight I could not touch my toes. I could barely do a pull-up and could only do about 20 push-ups — not very good by any standard of measurement. Still, people were cautioning me that weight training would make me tight and slow. After four months of a program, I had gained 15 pounds. I could touch my toes; in fact I could put my palms flat on the ground. I now could do 10 pull-ups and 50 push-ups and was noticeably faster. I could also now put my hand over the rim in basketball, where before I had been barely able to touch the rim.

Naturally I was questioning the myths. In fact, everything that both the coaches and many experts were saying was just the opposite of what had happened. I gained muscle, got more explosive, more flexible and faster. I realized that I was onto something and I needed to find out more. Thus began a magical mystery tour of trying out new training methods and ideas — a process that continues today.

The concept and application of strength training has evolved over the years

Following conventional wisdom of the time, there was no thought of weight training in season. Since I participated in three sports, the only time available to lift was after track ended in the spring until the start of football practice in September. The next off-season, which was before my freshman year in college, I was able to gain another 20 pounds and increase my explosiveness. I realize now in retrospect that some of this was normal growth and development coupled with the hard work. Directed work during a growth spurt when the body is secreting anabolic hormones like crazy is an optimum time to make gains. This is a clear message to all those high school age athletes who are seeking the magic bullet of supplementation. A good sound diet coupled with a well-designed training program during a growth spurt will yield spectacular results.

After my freshman football season at Fresno State College, there was no formal off-season program. We were instructed to be in shape for spring practice. Essentially we were on our own. We had one of the first Universal Gym multi-station weight machines and a few free weights. Naturally, since the machine was convenient and easy, that is what I used as my primary mode of training. I found immediately that my strength increased rapidly. In fact, I remember remarking to a friend that I could lift a lot more because I did not have to balance and control the weight. I quickly gained more muscle bulk. Now instead of feeling more explosive, I felt bulky and slower, but I thought that was ok because everyone else was doing it. The first day of spring practice, I pulled a hamstring — my first experience with anything like that. In retrospect, it had a lot to do with the type of lifting I was doing. Of course, I did not relate the two at the time.

In setting out to design my program in preparation for my sophomore year, I realized that I must get off the machines and do more work with free weights if I was going to develop the strength necessary to be a better football player. I had heard of a man named Alvin Roy who originally had worked with a high school in Louisiana and then with the LSU football program when they had won the national championship in 1958. He had worked with Billy Cannon, the Heisman trophy winner, and Jim Taylor who went on to star with the Green Bay Packers — both of whom were fast, explosive and agile. The things I read he was doing made a lot of sense. Through my high school football coach, I found out that he was now with the San Diego Chargers as their strength coach. As far as I know; he was the first strength coach in professional football and probably one of the first at any level. He had a book on their training program, which my high school coach lent me. I followed the programs down to the letter. It was a varied program that involved squatting, Olympic lifting movements, as well as functional isometric contractions. I saw improved results in terms of speed and explosiveness. The drawback was that I struggled to gain weight on the Charger program. Looking back, it was just too much work for my maturity level. Also, it was later revealed that the players on the Chargers had free access to anabolic steroids, which greatly enhanced their work capacity. There was no rest or recovery days built into the program, which at the time I thought was ok, but I now realize was a big mistake because I was always sore. The lesson to be learned here is that it is not advisable to blindly copy someone else's program unless you know all the factors and ingredients of the program.

Through articles in *Strength and Health* and watching the track team at Fresno State weight train, I quickly realized that the sport of track and field was very advanced in the use of weight training. Herb Elliot, who dominated the mile up through the Rome Olympics, and his coach, Percy Cerruty, made extensive use of strength training. Perry O'Brien, the first man to throw 60 feet in the shot put, was an avid weight trainer. He was fast enough to lead off a sprint relay, so it obviously did not slow him down! Dallas Long, the first man to throw over sixty-five feet, and Randy Matson, the first man to throw over 70, were all avid weight trainers. Lynn Davies, the 1964 Olympic Long Jump Champion, was able to significantly improve his speed. Russ Hodge, who broke the world record in the decathlon in the early sixties, made extensive use of weight training in his program. Chuck Coker, the coach at Occidental College in Los Angeles, was a pioneer in the implementation of weight training in Track and Field. In college it was the track team, especially the field event people under the direction of Coach Red Estes, who extensively used strength training — not the football team. Larry Alexander, a high jumper on the track team, had thoroughly studied the Russian high jump training methods used by Valeri Brummel, the world record holder at the time. Larry was kind enough to share his ideas with me. Brummel's program made extensive use of a variety of strength training exercises and jumping exercises that we would later call plyometrics. Larry also introduced me to *Track Technique,* a magazine devoted to presenting the latest training methods in track & field. These articles laid out a systematic approach as well as reasons for the drills and exercises. I find the information published in the early to mid sixties as timely today as it was then. It is no wonder that I found that when I worked out with the track athletes, I got my best results from my strength training program. The basic problem with all the programs that I used throughout college was a complete lack of any consideration for recovery. We went heavy on legs as often as three times a week, in addition to running every day, which never allowed our legs to recover. I thought a sore back and dead legs were just a normal part of the training. Fortunately or unfortunately, depending on how you look at it, we did not try to lift in season or during spring practice, which actually served as a break. The problem with no workouts in season is that every off-season, I was essentially starting over again. I questioned this because I saw the track athletes lifting throughout their season with no ill effects. In fact, the shot putters would often lift the day of the meet. Little did I realize that this was a portent of things to come.

The sport of track and field was the pioneer in the application of systematic strength training to improve sport performance.

After graduating from Fresno State, I went to UCSB for my teaching certification. While there, I was fortunate to take a class with Sherman Button on conditioning athletes. He was ahead of his time with the material and concepts that he presented. It was a great class because of his comprehensive approach to conditioning built around weight training. The two textbooks for the class were especially helpful: Pat Oshea's book *Scientific Principles and Methods of Strength Training* and *Foundations of Conditioning* by Falls, Walls and Logan. As a class assignment, we had to design a yearlong comprehensive training program for our chosen sports. I put together a program for track and field that incorporated all components of training. It was an initial attempt at periodization, but most importantly, it forced me to look at weight training in a new light. I was now a coach, as well as an athlete. I was responsible for other people. I had to teach them skill and have them ready for competition, so I had to pay attention to the big picture. Strength was only one part of the equation, although a most important part.

That spring in my first track coaching assignment, I got the opportunity to coach one of the best athletes I have ever coached: Sam Cunningham. He became California State Champion in the shot put that year and also an All American football running back. He was 6'3" tall, weighed 225, and could run the 100 in 9.7, but by my thinking he was "weak " because he could not lift much weight in the weight room. Yet he had tremendous explosive power. This led me to begin to ask the question: How much strength is enough? (A question I continue to ask.)

In the fall of 1969, I began training for the decathlon. I did all my strength training with Curt Harper, a world class discus thrower. Working with Curt, we trained on a varied program that involved Olympic lifting and power lifting. I got very strong. The only problem was that the work in the weight room was not transferring into performance on the track and in the field. Once again I begin to question the whole place that weight training had in a program.

Three things led me to modify my approach:
1) The writing of Ken Dougherty in his books *Modern Track and Field* and *Track and Field Omnibook,* especially the latter. In these books, he discussed concepts that would later evolve into my thinking on special and specific strength.
2) Training for the decathlon in Santa Barbara gave me the opportunity to train with some of the greatest athletes in the world. I saw how they trained. It also gave me first hand exposure to the European methods of training that, up until that point, I had only read about. This exposure to the Europeans led me to question the traditional approach that we were taking. They seemed to spend less time in the weight room. When they did come to the weight room, they were not as strong as we were, but they seemed to be able to do a better job of expressing their strength. They engaged in more varied activities like jumping and all types of throws.
3) In the fall of 1971, Pat Matzdorf from the University of Wisconsin moved to Santa Barbara to train. He had broken the world record in the high jump that year. His strength training was different. Bill Perrin, the track coach at Wisconsin (and a real innovator), designed his program. It involved simulation training, which consisted of specific strength training exercises that worked on various parts of the whole jump using a variety of methods including weights and rubber tubing. He also utilized depth jumps in his training. This was my first exposure to a systematic application of plyometric training.

From 1969 to 1973, I coached at La Cumbre Junior High School in Santa Barbara, California. It was first hand experience working with growth and development in the pre-pubescent and pubescent male athlete. There was not much equipment, even free weights. The strength program consisted primarily of push-ups, pull-ups, dips, and rope climb. At this age, with the tremendous linear growth that was occurring, body weight exercises were very appropriate loading. I felt that the key objective was to lay a base of athletic fitness that they could harness when they went to high school. Although at the time I felt somewhat shortchanged that we did not have more weights, in retrospect I was on the right track.

Another key milestone in the evolution of my ideas on training in general and strength training in particular was the 1972 "AAU Learn by Doing Track and Field Clinic" in Sacramento, California. Many of the top track & field coaches in the country were in attendance. The opportunity to interact with them was invaluable. Two of the "Learn by Doing" stations were devoted to plyometric training that was new and revolutionary at the time. Each evening there were presentations by Polish triple jump coach Tadeusz Starzynski. He presented the whole spectrum of his training program for triple jumpers that had produced Joseph Schmidt, three-time Olympic gold medalist. It obviously involved a lot of jumping exercises, but it included medicine ball work and some very specific weight training. There was nowhere near the extent of weight training we were having our athletes do, and the weight training that was done was much more specific. This experience had profound influence on how I trained my athletes for explosive power from that time on. I immediately incorporated his concepts and ideas in my personal training, as well as with the athletes I was coaching. The results were tremendous increases in explosiveness and speed.

In 1973 to 1974, while attending graduate school at Stanford University, I also had the opportunity to coach the jumpers and decathletes. This gave me the opportunity to apply what I had learned with more mature male athletes. It was also an opportunity to work with Payton Jordan, the track coach at Stanford who was a pioneer in weight training. He had worked with a man named John Jesse who authored many books on strength training for sport. Jesse was way ahead of his time in the application of strength training to prevention and rehabilitation of injuries. Doctor Wesley Ruff, my adviser, encouraged me to do research in the area of strength and power training, which I found very helpful. This helped me to better understand the scientific reasons for the things that I was observing as a coach and experiencing as an athlete.

My time at Santa Barbara High School (1975-77) was my first experience working with female athletes. I did not make distinctions as to gender: they were athletes. They strength trained with the boys. In fact, we learned that the girls derived even more spectacular benefits than the boys and that they needed to continue their strength training throughout the season or the drop off would be dramatic. The strength training was an important part of the program regardless of the event.

Before the late 1970's there did not seem to be the distinctions between all the styles of lifting. You just put together an eclectic program. You were not labeled a free weight guy, an Olympic lifting guy or a HIT guy, and you trained athletes. Two things changed this: 1)The ascendancy of Olympic lifting in the late 1970s which I believe resulted from the spectacular gains made by the Bulgarian weight lifters. The Bulgarian methods were thoroughly detailed by Carl Miller in his book *Olympic Lifting Training Manual*. The Olympic lifting movements had always played a major role in weight training for improving sport performance, but things seemed to change in the late seventies. There was an attempt to blindly copy Olympic lifting training protocols without any apparent regard to it's relationship to the whole training program. Just because an Olympic lifter, who does nothing but lift, is able to lift up to five times a day does not mean that a football player or a basketball player who has to run and jump and do other training should attempt multiple lifting sessions in a day. Olympic lifting for sport performance is a means to an end. If you are an Olympic weight lifter then it is as end in itself, because those lifts are the performance standard. 2) In the mid 1970's a new machine-oriented system was invented by Arthur Jones: the Nautilus system which was based on eccentric loading and one set to failure. It was not that these were the first machines, but they were the first machines that were marketed with a training system and philosophy to back them up. It appealed to the American mentality of instant gratification. It was hard work, but it was over rather quickly. In addition, because of the eccentric emphasis it was possible to gain hypertrophy rather quickly which appealed to American football.

Things began to change rapidly with the advent of the full-time professional "Strength Coach." In the seventies very few colleges had strength coaches. If they did, most of their attention was centered on football. In professional sport there were few full-time strength coaches. In 1976 Bob Ward, who was the track coach at Fullerton College in California, was hired by the Dallas Cowboys. He had a full time year-round program that was backed by management so that the players had to comply. This was the exception, not the norm. Superior talent and genetics continued to prevail even into the late 1980's. Not all the teams in professional football had full-time strength and conditioning coaches. The advent of the strength coach in college and professional sport was like a good news, bad news joke. The good news was that now there would be someone who whose sole responsibility was to condition the athletes. The bad news was that with the exception of those who had a track and field background, they seldom got out of the weight room.

In 1985 I began my foray into professional sports with the Chicago White Sox and the Bulls as an assistant to Al Vermeil. I was surprised to see the old myths and misconceptions that I thought had been forgotten were still bring there. One would have thought that by 1985 with the success that athletes had enjoyed world wide with comprehensive conditioning programs that the coaches and athletes would have embraced this training as an opportunity to better themselves. But, I believe that as there had been little emphasis on training in professional basketball and baseball, the attitude on the part of the coaches was let them play—those who are talented will succeed and those who are not will fall by the wayside. I kept hearing that basketball and baseball were different. Don't lift heavy because it will hurt your shooting. The trainer told me that pitchers should not lift overhead because it would hurt their shoulder. When I stated that they lifted their arm overhead when they pitched, I was told I didn't understand the game.

In 1987 I took over as Director of Conditioning for the Chicago White Sox. This gave me the opportunity to put together a systematic comprehensive program in professional sport. No one in professional baseball had a systematic year-round program. In order to make it work I decided that we needed to make the program more specific to the demands of the sport of baseball. It needed to include more work on balance and proprioception, more work on rotation. I was very influenced by Dr. Lois Klatt, head of the Human Performance Lab at Concordia University in River Forest, Illinois and the book *Total Body Training*, by Bob Gajda and Robert Dominguez. Through their influence and working closely with Gary Gray, PT, from Adrian Michigan, I gradually moved away from weight training to the concept of strength training. Weight training is one method of strength training. In order to train a complete athlete, it is necessary to utilize all methods available to achieve the desired goal. What evolved was a functional strength training program that was adapted to the multi-plane demands of the sport of baseball as well as the unique demands of the specific positions. The program was based on biomechanical analysis so that the movements we were training were more specific. Pitchers had a specific program and catchers had a specific program, rather than one program for all. All these programs had all components linked so that what was done with speed and agility training was related to balance and proprioception work which in turn was related to the strength training work. My goal with the White Sox was to create a model that would work in any sport. I was fortunate to be able to use the resources available to work toward accomplishing this task. We were able to achieve good results with the White Sox both in terms of measurable improvements of speed and power, as well as significant reduction of injuries.

> *The strength coach is a relatively recent phenomenon in the world of sports*

Gary Gray enabled me to take a major step forward with his input. Gary is a brilliant, creative individual who has a unique eye for human movement that enables him to think outside the box. Movement is multi-joint, multi-plane, and involves balance and proprioception. He got me to think past the muscle and look closely at the movement.

Monkey see, monkey do syndrome. If it is good for them and they just won the national championship, then it is good for us. There is a prevalent attitude that the greatest testament for a piece of equipment or a particular training method is the affirmation of winning. What I have seen through my experience is that success is often achieved in spite of, not because of the training and that superior talent and genetics sometimes prevail. A good sound training program is not based on equipment or personalities, but on sound scientific training principles. We need to consider what is really "high tech." I got a call recently from a friend who had just visited a new high tech training facility. They had a machine for everything. Everything was connected to a computer. What is more high tech—the machine or the body? I have come to the realization that the body is the ultimate high tech machine. The farther away we get from the body, the less specific the training.

Where are we going? What have we learned? The key is the nervous system. That is what Sam Cunningham was trying to tell me in my first year of coaching. What was most important was not that he could not lift more weight. It is how you can recruit and fire the muscles in a coordinated pattern that is most important. Strength training is about neural drive; it is training the command and control system. That is why it is so important to train movements, not muscles! This is where we have to go in order to progress to do a better job of integrating strength training: make it specific in order to develop athleticism. ◆

Everything in Balance

Michael Jordan had it. Emmitt Smith has it. Serena Williams has it. What is it? Balance. It is the single most important component of athletic ability because it underlies all movement. It is a relatively simple concept, but can have many complex applications.

For example, a relatively simple activity such as sprinting, when seen from a balance perspective, is highly complex. At speeds in excess of 11 meters per second, the sprinter must alternate balancing on one leg and then the other in less than one tenth of a second. Try losing and regaining your balance in less than one tenth of a second and see how difficult a skill it is.

In athletics, balance does not work in isolation. Therefore, it should not be thought of as an isolated component. For example, coordination and agility depend on a well developed sense of balance. In fact, balance is a component of all movement whether that movement is dominated by strength, speed, flexibility, or stamina.

To better understand this concept, take another look at an activity you are training for from the perspective of the role of balance in that activity. Problems that seem to be related to strength, speed, flexibility, or skill can in fact be balance-related and are simply manifested as a lack of strength, speed, flexibility, or skill. Poor balance can also lead to poor technical or skill development, which often results in injury.

Balance in Motion

Because of the traditional definition, we tend to think of balance as static—as in a person standing straight for a period of time. However, in function balance is dynamic. Because an athlete is constantly moving, balance entails the body repeatedly losing and regaining control of its center of gravity in its attempt to perform efficient movement. Additionally, there is a continual reaction to other external forces such as the playing surface, opponents, and the ball.

Maintaining this state of dynamic equilibrium requires total systemic involvement with feedback from the ocular, vestibular, kinesthetic, and auditory senses. Overall, our goal must be to develop good balance in motion—not in a still position. To do this we must train, test, and rehab balance in motion, not in stillness.

Balance also has an integral relationship with the concept of the Performance Paradigm (see page 11). This concept states that it is impossible to appropriately reduce and subsequently produce force without balance.

Whether it's on the balance beam or the basketball court, dynamic balance is a key to all athletic endeavors.

In other words, the ability to reduce force at the right time, at the right joint, in the right plane, in the right direction, for the right activity is highly balance-dependent. The inability to do all of the above will result in movement that is awkward and not necessarily in the direction desired.

Conceptually, it may be helpful to think of balance as occurring in two zones: the Inner Zone and the Outer Zone. With Inner Zone Balance, body weight and center of gravity are directly over the ground reaction force to our center of gravity. It is the traditional static standing position, and it is not highly functional. It serves only as a starting position for more complex and demanding drills.

Outer Zone Balance refers to how far outside your Inner Zone you can reach or step and still retain balance. The point at which you lose control of your balance for that particular activity is the Balance Threshold. At any point past this Threshold, balance is lost, which leads to inefficient movement and wasted energy. If you lose your balance but do not fall over, it is still regarded as lost balance. Using energy to try to regain your balance is using energy inefficiently, because it is not directly related to your goal.

What we are seeking is a functional threshold—a point at which motion is productive. This threshold must be constantly stressed with functional movement patterns to improve balance.

It is important to understand what is affecting balance in order to be able to effectively train balance. Essentially it is anything that manipulates the force that we have to balance against. It could be your opponent, the effects of gravity, the angle of the ground/surface, the direction of movement, your arms and legs, the wind, a weight, or a stretch cord.

Training Balance

Balance is improved through exposure to a variety of different sensory conditions in a safe, controlled environment. To design a functional balance training program, we must increase proprioceptive demand in normal training activities. In selecting balance exercises, use the following criteria:
- The exercise must be safe.
- It must be challenging.
- It must stress multiple planes of motion.
- It must incorporate a multi-sensory approach.
- It must be derived from a fundamental movement skill and applied directly to a sport skill.

Balance must be developed in a progressive manner. The goal is to continually increase awareness of the Balance Threshold by creating instability. The following progression is appropriate for both Inner Zone and Outer Zone balance activities.

1. Begin with a bilateral stance (two legs).
2. Progress to a unilateral stance (one leg), first using the arms as a counterbalance, then without using arms.
3. Attempt exercise with eyes closed.
4. Try varied surfaces that make balance more difficult.
5. Incorporate different apparatus.
6. Progress to dynamic activities.
7. Increase the range of motion.
8. Increase the speed.
9. Try activities that require reaction.
10. Increase the external kinesthetic stimulus.

The volume of work completed on balance should be low, although it should be incorporated into the workout routine on a daily basis. For balance work to be most effective it demands the highest degree of intensity and concentration. Thus it is most efficient and beneficial to train balance as a part of the warm-up or between drills during practice.

Sample Exercises

The following sample exercises are intended for use with various sports for both training and rehabilitation. They are all simple activities that can be easily incorporated into the daily routine. Use your imagination and knowledge and invent your own balance exercises and activities.

Leaning Tower — Sway anterior/posterior and medial/lateral.

Hurdle Walk — Step over hurdle and hold position for a count of one-thousand-one, then step over the next hurdle and repeat with the opposite leg. To increase difficulty, close the eye of the leg that is stepping over the hurdle.

Scramble Up — Start from a prone position and scramble up to a balance standing position as quickly as possible. To increase the difficulty, perform the exercise with the eyes closed.

Ninety-Degree Jumps — Jump and turn 90 degrees in the air. Land and jump and turn 90 degrees in the opposite direction back to the starting position. Jump and turn 180, then 270, and finally 360 degrees. Eyes open. Eyes closed.

Red Light/Green Light — Stop on one leg each time and hold a balance position in response to a random signal.

Rhythmic Balance Exercises — Use a metronome or music to govern the rate of a particular balance activity.

It is also effective to use an oscillating balance beam, a K-board, a BAPS Board, mini tramp, gymnic balls, or a foam block to perform balance activities. Don't get too hung up on equipment though, and remember that the body is still the highest-tech training equipment one can use.

Testing Balance

It is necessary to effectively test balance in order to train balance. Testing is best accomplished using functional movements that provide real feedback that the body can immediately interpret and use. It is important to test both Inner Zone and Outer Zone Balance.

To test the effect of the various sensory systems, perform testing with and without those systems. For example, to test the effect of the ocular system test with both the eyes open and closed. Testing will give an objective measure of improvement. The important aspect of testing, just as in training, is that it must relate to the activity that you are preparing for.

Overall, in testing and training balance, remember to keep your sport-specific goals in mind. The goal of balance training for most athletes is not to be able to walk a tightrope or ride a unicycle. But it may be to hit a 10-foot jumper balancing on one leg or increase the velocity of a fastball by having more control of the back leg during the wind-up. The key is determining when balance will most affect performance.

For further information on testing we refer you to *Lower Extremity Functional Profile* by Gary Gray with Team Reaction (Wynne Marketing, Adrian, Mich: 1994). ◆

The Core Of the Matter

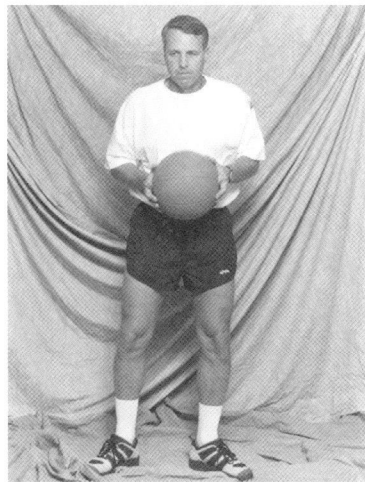 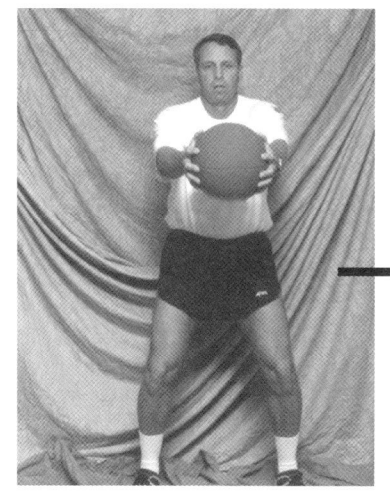 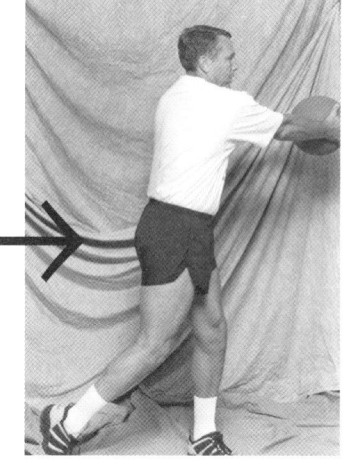

Figure One: Tight Rotation Starting Position

Figure Two: Wide Rotation

The core is the center of the body, a hub where trunk and ground forces converge and are modulated. It is where the body's center of gravity is located. Yet it is often neglected in the training of competitive athletes.

Anatomically, the core consists of the muscles of the hips, abdomen, and lower back. The core includes some of the largest muscles of the body. For certain sports, the core can be extended to include the upper back and neck due to the role these muscles play in postural alignment, balance, and support of the head.

Gravity, Posture & Balance

One of the reasons why the core is so important is because the structural integrity of the body depends on it. Controlling gravity, posture, and balance are all major factors in athletic performance, and they are all greatly affected by the muscles of the core.

When standing, the body's center of gravity is located approximately two inches below the navel, in the middle of the core muscles. In any sporting activity, we require the body to overcome, or at the very least neutralize, the effects of gravity.

Gravity also has a profound effect on posture, which is controlled by the core muscles. Through stabilization, the core muscles help maintain good posture, and they do this by being continually active. We tend to think of posture as a rigid and static position relating to postural analysis in a posture grid. In practice though, posture is highly dynamic not only in athletics, but in the activities of daily life.

Control of the core is also essential for balance because all movement is controlled and modulated by the stronger, slower muscles surrounding the athlete's center of gravity. This is why coaches emphasize watching an opponent's navel while playing defense. In the martial arts, control of the center-or Ki is an essential element.

The basic principle that we can derive from the above points is that in order to ensure proper functional strength development, it is necessary to develop core strength before extremity strength. This is not static strength, but dynamic strength that allows the body to move efficiently through a variety of positions.

Athletes in a training program tend to work the arms and the legs and ignore the core area or leave it until the end of the workout, where it is short-changed. If the extremities are strong and the core is weak, then there will not be enough force generated in those extremities to produce efficient movement. A weak core is a fundamental cause of inefficient movement—as well as the source of many injuries, and this weakness will be particularly magnified in a fatigued state.

The core is the center of the body where all movement is modulated.

Functional Training

To actually train the core, it is important to use multi-plane movements that are functional and synergistic. Most people think of training the core through sit-ups and back extensions. However, this only works one aspect of the core: the muscles that control trunk flexion and extension. This approach leads to unbalanced development, which may cause back injuries because the muscles that support the spine in multi-plane movements are ignored.

To be functional, the movements must include rotational

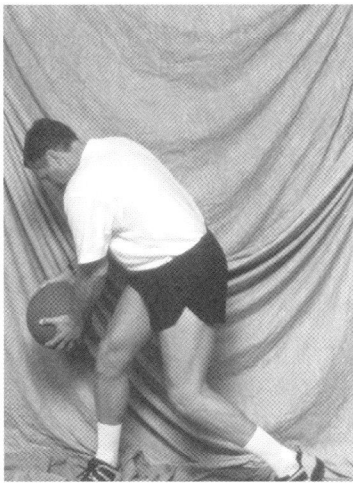
Figure Three: Chop to the Waist

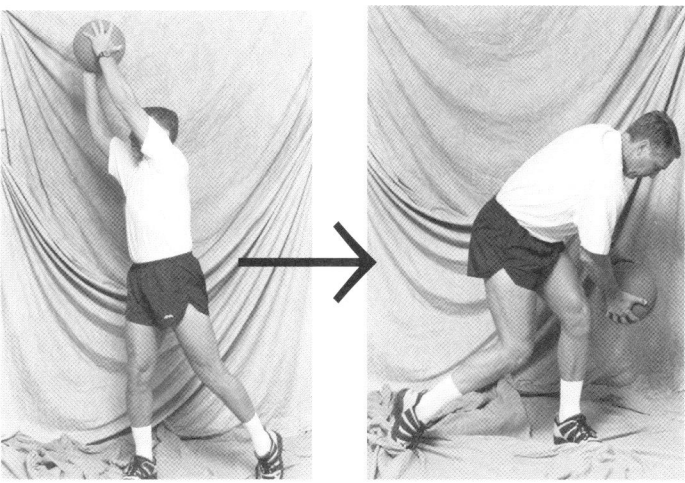
Figure Four Chop to the Knee

movements and diagonal patterns in addition to flexion and extension. We must get away from trying to isolate specific muscles of the core and integrate all involved muscles into functional patterns. To achieve optimum performance, it is necessary to condition and prepare the whole body as a link system with all its parts working together. The core is perhaps the most essential link in the kinetic chain because of its function and location.

Along the same lines, it is important to understand that those exercises performed in the standing position are more functional than those performed while seated or lying down. In the supine, prone, or seated position, the pelvis is fixed. Therefore, it is not allowed to rotate normally and transfers forces artificially to areas not designed to take the stress that is imposed. The goal is not to isolate, but to integrate muscles into functional movement patterns. The most functional posture, in order to allow for hip rotation and to take full advantage of the effects of gravity, is the standing position.

The principles that apply to training other parts of the body also apply to the core. To properly train the core muscles, they must be worked through a full range of motion, they must be overloaded, and adequate time between workouts must be allowed for recovery. Due to their slow-twitch nature, these muscles can tolerate a large workload and recover quickly. The movements that work the muscles of the core are trunk flexion and extension (bending forward and back in the sagittal plane), lateral flexion (bending to the side in the frontal plane), trunk rotation (turning side to side in the transverse plane), and combinations of these movements that involve multi-plane functional patterns.

The following exercises address all these movements in a functional continuum. They incorporate different postures that can be done solo or with a partner, and they only require a medicine ball or the athlete's weight. It is important to realize that exercises in the lying position where the pelvis is fixed are less functional, and therefore should occupy a smaller proportion of the training time. These exercises are not the only ones that you should use, but provide examples to get you started.

Lying Posture

Leg Raise — Place hands under the pelvis for stabilization and to take the curve out of the low back. Slightly bend the knees. Raise and lower the legs 18 to 24 inches.

Lower Ab Sit Up — Same position as the previous exercise but bring the knees back toward the chest and shoot the feet toward the ceiling.

Curl Up — Bend knees with feet flat on the floor. Fold arms across chest and keep the chin tucked in. Curl trunk off the ground, imagining that you are lifting one vertebra at a time until the trunk is flexed 30 degrees off the floor.

Crunch — Bend knees with the thighs perpendicular to the ground and the foreleg parallel to the ground. Curl the trunk off the ground, attempting to bring the chest to the thigh.

Twister — Same as previous exercise but lock the hands behind the head. Curl up and twist, touching the right elbow to the outside of the left thigh and the left elbow to the outside of the right thigh.

Seated Posture

Russian Twist — Seated, bend the knees and keep the feet flat on the floor and the upper body inclined back at a 45-degree angle. Extend arms out in front of chest with palms together. Rotate trunk to the right and to the left.

American Twist — While seated, position the legs in a v-sit, flat on the floor and the torso upright. Hold arms close to the body, with one hand over the other. Beginning with the hands on the ground off the left hip, rotate trunk to the right and back again to the left. This rotation should be in tight circles close to the body.

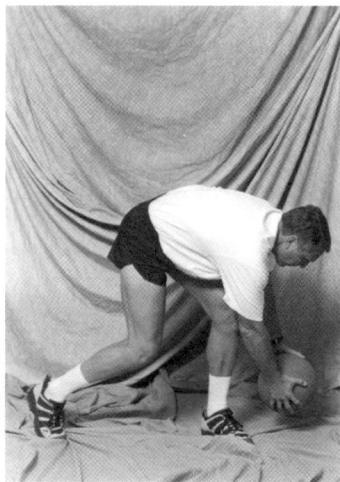

Figure Five: Chop to the Ankle

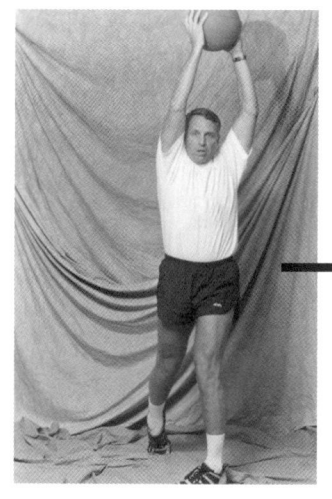

Figure Six-A: Woodchopper Top Position

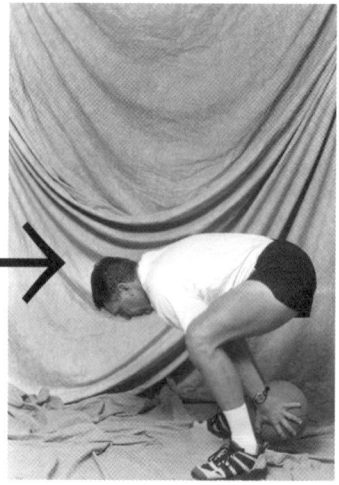

Figure Seven-B: Woodchopper Bottom Position

Standing Posture

All of the following exercises should be done with the feet shoulder-width apart or slightly wider. The knees should be slightly flexed.

Tight Rotation — With the ball held directly in front of the navel close to the body, rotate as far around to the right as possible and then immediately rotate to the left. Be sure to unlock the hips as you rotate. (See Figure One for starting position.)

Wide Rotation — Same as the previous exercise but now hold the arms extended out from the waist and swing the ball around in a wide arc. (Figure Two)

Chop to the Waist — Start with the ball held overhead off to one side. Chop down and across to the opposite side hip. Repeat 10 times for each side. (Figure Three)

Chop to the Knee — Start with the ball held overhead off to one side. Chop down and across to the opposite knee. Repeat 10 times for each side. (Figure Four)

Chop to the Ankle — Start with the ball held overhead off to one side. Chop down and across to the opposite side ankle. Repeat five times for each side. Be sure to stand up completely after each repetition and reach as high as possible with the ball. (Figure Five)

Woodchopper with a Twist — Start with the ball held directly overhead. Chop straight down between the legs. Straighten up and twist either right or left after each repetition and reach as high as possible with the ball. Repeat ten times with a twist at the top after each repetition, alternating twisting right and left. (Figure Six-A is Ending Position; Figure Six-B is Bottom Position)

Squat and Touch — Stand on one leg. With the opposite hand touch six points on the floor around the body. Be sure to return to a full standing position after each touch. When bending to touch, be sure to bend, flexing at the ankle, knee, and hip. (Figure Seven-A is Starting Position; Figure Seven-B is Touch Across; Figure Seven-C is Touch in Front)

Medicine Ball Partner Exercises

Medicine Ball Half Twist — Partners stand back to back one arm's distance apart. Twist to one side and pass the ball to the second partner who rotates around to the opposite side and passes back to the first partner. The ball moves around the outside of the two partners.

Medicine Ball Full Twist — Partners stand back to back one arm's distance apart. Twist to one side and pass the ball to the second partner's opposite side and that partner then turns the opposite way and passes back to the first partner. The ball moves in a figure eight pattern between the two partners.

Chop with a Push — One partner stands with the ball held overhead off to one side. The second partner pushes on the ball as the first partner chops down and across to the opposite side hip. Repeat 10 times for each side.

Rotation with a Push — The first partner holds the ball out with arms extended from the waist, while the second partner pushes the ball around in a wide arc. The action is repeated to the opposite side. Repeat 10 times for each side.

Medicine Ball Throws

These exercises are best done against a sturdy wall, although they can be done with a partner.

Overhead Throw — Stand one arm's distance away from the wall with the feet shoulder-width apart and arms extended straight overhead. Slightly flex the knees and bend back about 10 degrees and throw the ball against the wall while attempting to keep the arms as straight as possible. Catch the ball overhead and repeat 20 times.

Soccer Throw — Stand one and one-half arm's distance away from the wall with feet should-width apart and the arms bent behind the head. Slightly flex the knees, bend back about 10 degrees, and throw the ball against the wall while extending the

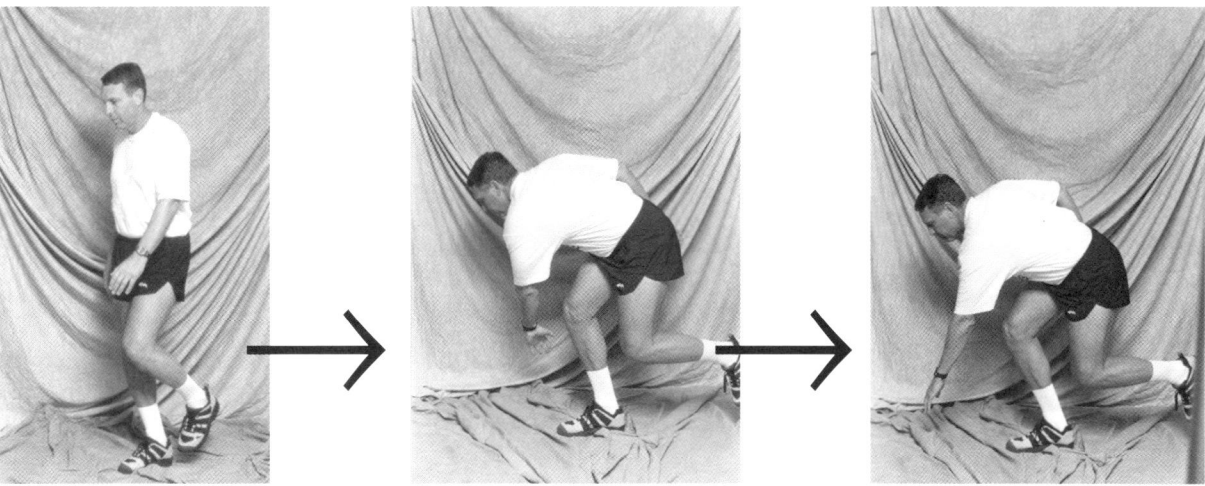

Figure Seven-B: Squat and Touch, Starting Position

Figure Seven-C: Squat and Touch, Touch Across

Figure Seven-C: Squat and Touch, Touch In Front

arms. Catch the ball and let momentum carry the ball back to the starting position. Immediately repeat 20 times.

Side To Side Throw — Stand about body height away from the wall with the feet slightly wider than shoulder-width apart. Start with the ball at waist height on one side of the body. Swing the ball to a point on the wall at waist height so that the ball is deflected off at an angle to the opposite side of the body. Let the weight of the ball twist the torso. Retrieve the ball and throw it back to the opposite side. Repeat 10 times for each side.

Down the Side Throw — Stand about body height away from the wall with feet slightly wider than shoulder width apart. Start with the ball at waist height on one side. Swing the ball to a point on the wall at waist height so that the ball hits directly outside the same side hip. Let the weight of the ball twist the torso and repeat the throw to the same side. Repeat the throwing motion 10 times for each side.

Around the Back Throw — Stand facing away from the wall about body height from the wall with feet slightly wider than shoulder width apart. Start with the ball at waist height on one side or the other. Swing the ball to a point on the wall at waist height so that the ball is deflected off at an angle to the opposite side. Let the weight of the ball twist the torso. Retrieve the ball, and throw it back to the opposite side. Repeat 10 times for each side.

Training Schedule

The muscles of the core can be trained daily by carefully mixing the movements and the exercises to stress different muscles each day and giving them adequate time to recover. A good sequence to use over a three-day period is:

Day One: Flexion and extension movements.
Day Two: Rotation, twisting, and chopping movements.
Day Three: Throws and catches.

Repeat this cycle again for the following three days, either repeating the same exercises or selecting different exercises that serve the same function. Take the seventh day off as a recovery day. A maximum of six to ten exercises can be completed in one session consisting of ten to 20 reps for each exercise.

Allocate 15 to 20 minutes daily for core work, although it will take less time after the technique of each exercise is learned. Rotations, twists, chopping, flexion, and extension movements are especially effective as a warm up for reactive ballistic exercise. The throws, however, should be done as a segment of the actual workout or as an actual workout in order to ensure high intensity and proper mechanics. ◆

Strength In Motion

It is an acknowledged fact that strength is an important factor in performance and rehabilitation. However, the concept of strength cannot be defined as simply the number of pounds lifted or number of repetitions completed. Strength has many different implications, depending on the specific sport or rehab situation, and it should be viewed as only one aspect of athletic performance.

Traditional strength training programs often fail to take into account how much strength is actually necessary and what types of strength are specifically needed for the given sport. According to John Jesse, a pioneer in the area of strength training and physical therapy, "Because strength is easier to develop than other qualities, athletes have spent more time improving strength rather than developing speed, timing, balance, and other skills that would put their strength to greater use in performance."

How strong do you have to be to hit a five-ounce baseball or to serve a tennis ball? Does it take a different type and amount of strength to throw a 16-pound shot as compared to playing an offensive line position in football? Will the increased strength improve your performance or enhance rehabilitation? The key to answering these questions involves thinking about the application of the strength in the given situation.

Strength has many different applications depending on the specific sport or rehab situation.

Defining Strength

Strength is the ability to exert force, period — without any time constraints. Power is the ability to exert maximal force within the shortest time frame possible. What we usually call strength, as it relates to sports performance, is actually power. Almost all sport performance demands high force production in short periods of time, usually in .25 seconds or less. It also demands the subsequent ability to stop or decelerate that force in an equally short period of time. Therefore, athletic performance can be defined as the constant interplay between force production and force reduction, both of which usually occur over very brief time spans.

It is also helpful to think of strength as a continuum, with General Strength at one end, Specific Strength at the other, and Transitional Strength in between. This approach allows for a broad performance spectrum that transfers to sport performance.

General Strength consists of traditional weight training exercises and other resistance methods that do not seek to imitate specific sports skills. Traditional weight lifting and body weight exercises are examples of this classification. Specificity of movement with regard to mechanics and speed is a low priority.

Transitional Strength is movement with resistance that incorporates the joint dynamics of a sport's skills. The speed component is higher and movement is more specific than General Strength exercises. Most medicine ball exercises and plyometrics exercise are examples of this classification.

Specific Strength involves a high degree of specificity with regard to both mechanics and speed while imitating the specific joint action of the desired skill. There is very little distinction between special and specific strength. When the distinction does occur, it is a matter of emphasis and degree due to differences in training age, level of ability, time of the training year, and the sport. (See Table One for examples).

Application of Strength

Somehow the misconception has arisen that strength training equals weight training. This is very limiting and does not allow for much latitude in designing the strength training aspects of a total conditioning program. Another misconception is that strength must be measured as the amount of weight lifted or force registered on an isokinetic dynamometer. Experience has shown that increasing measurable strength does not necessarily transfer to improved sports performance or more effective rehabilitation. Strength is better thought of in terms of functional strength, i.e., the strength that can be applied to performance. For example, a leg extension and a leg curl are single-joint exercises which provide measurable strength, but not much functional strength. However, a single-leg squat is a multi-joint exercise which involves balance and provides functional strength.

Similarly, strength training should be thought of as one of many means to an end—not as an end in itself. In other words, the mode of strength training should not be emphasized to the exclusion of the ultimate objective of the training program: improved performance in a specific sport. Strength training must be considered within the context of the sport and the specific needs of the athlete. The entire conditioning program must be synergistic, meaning that the whole is greater than the sum of its parts. No one aspect of training should receive emphasis at the expense of another.

Choosing Functional Exercises

A basic principle of functional strength development is the use of body weight before that of external resistance. The athlete should be able to handle body weight in exercises like pull-ups, dips, step-ups, etc., before attempting to lift external weights. This approach develops balance, proprioception, the synergistic muscles,

TABLE ONE: Strength Continuum Examples

Sport/Skill	General Strength	Transitional Strength	Specific Strength
Tennis Serve	Dumbbell Pullover	Two Arm Medicine Ball Throw	One Arm Medicine Ball Throw
Basketball	Squat with Weight	Body Weight Squat	Squat Jumps
Track Sprinter	Lunge	Bounding	Towing
Football Offensive Line	Bench Press	Heavy Blocking Dummy	Two Man Sled
Baseball Pitcher	Pullover	Two Arm Medicine Ball Throw	Throw 12-oz. Ball From Cocked Position

and, most importantly, it will ensure proper progression and preparation for the more specific work to follow. For the younger developing athlete, it also addresses the concern of when to begin weight training, which should occur only after the developing athlete can handle his or her own body weight. Remember that the body is the ultimate free weight!

This leads us to another principle: performance and function are the result of a series of integrated and coordinated movements. Therefore, movements should be trained as opposed to training isolated muscles and hoping to transfer that strength to a functional movement. For example, Knee Flexion/Extension can be combined with Hip Flexion/Extension to ensure the development of functional strength. A step-up, a single-leg squat, or a traditional squat are preferable to leg extensions, leg curls, or multi-hip machines that isolate the respective muscles. In addition, training movements are much more efficient in terms of utilizing training time and facilities than training isolated muscles.

Traditionally, the focus of strength training has been on force production. There is an increasing realization, however, that most performance errors and injuries occur during the force reduction phase of movement. Therefore, the importance of this phase must also be emphasized. For example, when an athlete performs a squat, he or she should not just emphasize the ascending motion, but must also concentrate on the descending motion within the exercise. Maintaining a constant interplay between force production and force reduction will result in injury-free and efficient sport performance.

The fundamental criterion for selecting a weight training exercise is that it should incorporate diagonal-rotational patterns which are multi-plane and multi-joint. This concept effectively eliminates those machines that are designed to isolate muscles and work in single-joint, single-plane movements. Many standard weight machines and isokinetic devices are non-functional, I believe, because the type of strength developed is not readily transferred to sport performance and can thus interfere with coordination patterns and cause strength imbalances that predispose the athlete to injury.

Among the best methods of increasing functional strength are dumbbell and free-weight training because they allow for unilateral work that can be performed in multi-joint, multi-plane, diagonal-rotational patterns. These types of exercises are functional and measurable, not in terms of pounds lifted but in application to function. Dumbbell and free-weight training develop balance, stabilization, joint proprioception, and kinesthesis.

Olympic Lifts

There is a school of thought among strength coaches that has placed an inordinate emphasis on the Olympic-style lifts as the primary focus of strength training programs. This practice is based on the fallacious logic that Olympic lifters are the strongest athletes in the world, and this type of strength has direct application to other sports. Olympic weight lifting is a sport unto itself. The two Olympic lifts—the Clean and Jerk, the Snatch and their various derivatives—train the movements necessary to achieve success in Olympic weight lifting. Those movements produce very high power production in the vertical plane, but involve no rotational-diagonal component. This leads me to question the application of Olympic lifts in other sports.

Another factor to consider is that Olympic lifters do not have to do anything but lift. They are not practicing to perform in another sport or to acquire other skills and conditioning. They have a very narrow performance spectrum and only one focus, which is to gain as much strength as possible in the two lifts required to be successful in their sport. Therefore, blindly copying the training patterns and intensities that are used by Olympic lifters can have many negative over-training connotations for the athlete preparing for another sport.

In addition, Olympic lifts require high skill component,

which must be mastered in order to minimize the risk of injury and maximize the training benefit. Fatigue from a preceding workout can compromise the skill of performing the Olympic lifts, and incorrect technique can predispose the athlete to injury — especially to the lower back. It does not seem appropriate to spend the time mastering these skills when training time is limited and other strength training activities could accomplish the same objective with less risk.

That is not to say that Olympic lifting has no application. Rather, it is important to understand its limitations and to carefully consider why you want to incorporate these movements into a strength training program. They should be incorporated as a part of a program rather than be its focal point.

I realize that many of the thoughts expressed in this chapter differ from conventional wisdom. Hopefully this has stimulated you to take another look at strength training and its role in conditioning and rehabilitation. ◆

Strength By Design

For some strength coaches, it's the best part of the job. For others, it's the worst. But, for all strength coaches, it's critical to their athletes' success. I'm referring to program design — the time spent away from our athletes and at our desks plotting and strategizing the everyday workouts. Even if you've been a strength coach for many years, this can be one of the most challenging parts of your job. There are so many factors to consider, including the sport, the athletes, and your resources.

In addition, much of the information available on the topic is littered with a confusing barrage of fads, myths, misconceptions, half truths, and lies. In this chapter, I hope to cut through some of this confusion by providing practical pointers that will lead you step-by-step through the development of a strength-training program — whether it's for a new athlete, for a new sport, or to redesign an ineffective program.

The Principles

To get off on the right foot with your program, you need to understand and embrace those principles of strength training that are sound. They can be summed up in the following six points:

Develop sport-specific strength — This is the most important principle and is also usually the goal of any strength-training program. Except for competitive weight-lifters, the goal is NOT to increase the athlete's ability to lift heavier weights. The goal is to develop strength that the athlete can use in his or her sport.

Strength training is a spectrum of activities — This includes more than lifting weights. Under the umbrella of strength training, I include body-weight exercise, core training, plyometric training, free-weight training, machine training, Olympic lifting, and power lifting.

Train movements, not muscles — The central nervous system (CNS) is the command station that controls and directs all movement. The CNS calls for pre-programmed patterns of movement that can be modified in countless ways to react appropriately to gravity, ground-reaction forces, and momentum. Each activity is subjected to further refinements and adjustments by feedback from the body's proprioceptors. This process ensures optimal neuromuscular control and efficiency of function. For this reason, it's critical that we think of movement not as an isolated event that occurs in one plane of motion, but as a complex event that involves synergists, stabilizers, neutralizers, and antagonists all working together. Movement does not occur in the anatomical position, and choosing exercises that isolate specific muscles does not appropriately address dynamic, multi-dimensional strength development. Movement occurs in reaction to gravity, ground reaction forces, and momentum and must be trained as such.

Designing a strength training program specific to a sport depends on the application of basic principles.

Train core before extremity strength — A strong, stable core consisting of the the hip, abdomen, and low back is the cornerstone of a strength-training program. Without a strong, stable core, loading the extremities will be very risky and limited by the lack of core strength. The core works as a transmitter, transferring force from the lower to the upper extremity and vice versa.

Train body weight before external resistance — This entails being able to overcome gravitational loading in traditional body-weight exercises like the push-up, pull-up, and body-weight squat before adding weights. This type of work will help to strengthen the tendons and ligaments as well as the muscles in preparation for external loading. It will also ensure good joint stability.

Train strength before strength endurance — Traditionally, strength training programs have started with circuit training in order to build a foundation of strength endurance. But, in order to endure strength, it is first necessary to build strength. Only when a base of strength has been established can you work to add an endurance component.

Asking Questions

Using these principles as a guide, the next step in designing a program requires asking questions of yourself, your coaches, and your athletes. The first group of questions includes the following: What do you hope to achieve with a strength training program? What are the team's goals? What are the individual's goals? How can strength training help realize these goals? The answers to these questions should be based on three factors: the sport, the athlete, and the environment.

The Sport

A tennis player should have a different program than a football player. In fact, a quarterback should have a different program than a lineman. To figure out how to make the strength training program match the sport and position, consider these next questions:
- What are the strength requirements of the sport and position?
- What muscle groups are used?
- What are the movement requirements?
- What is the direction of the application of force?
- What is the range of movement?
- What kind of resistance does the athlete have to overcome?
- Is added muscle mass needed for armor and protection?
- What are the common injuries?

The Athlete

In looking at the individual athlete, carefully consider growth and development factors as well as previous injuries and gender. Questions here include the following:

- Has the athlete gone through puberty? While there is no doubt that the pre-pubescent athlete can weight train (research and practical experience have shown no ill effects from weight training), I tend to modify programs for younger athletes. My rule is to avoid any heavy loading of the spine until after puberty. Thus, I limit the amount of overhead work that a young athlete does, and I put the emphasis on body-weight exercises. This will serve as excellent preparation to safely move forward on the strength continuum after puberty.
- Is the athlete an early or late developer? Biological and chronological age are often quite different, so it's important to take into account an athlete's maturity as well as his or her age. Cognitive and emotional development should also be considered, as they are quite important to the athlete's ability to accept coaching and learn exercises and routines.
- What is the athlete's medical history? Along with addressing any past injuries, carefully evaluate any significant postural defects. Problems with posture, including gait mechanics, must be addressed before moving any further into a training program.
- What are the athlete's unique, individual qualities? Does he or she need to develop in an area that is slowing him or her down? If the athlete cannot do an exercise, find a simpler, more remedial exercise to substitute.
- If the athlete is female, does she lack a strength base? Because our culture encourages boys to participate in more physical activities, they often enter their first strength-training program with a base. Many girls, however, start sport programs with bodies that have experienced very little strength training. In addition, the female athlete typically has a smaller percentage of total body mass as muscle.

Therefore, strength training may be more important for the female athlete than the male. In fact, I feel strongly that the female athlete should begin strength training earlier than boys and continue strength training throughout the training year and her career. It has been my observation (albeit neither supported nor refuted by research) that the female athlete who begins a sound, well-rounded strength-training program before puberty tends to more easily maintain that strength base after puberty. Also, because the female matures earlier than the male, it is easier to begin strength training earlier.

The Environment

From a coaching and teaching perspective, it is important to take into consideration outside factors that will affect the strength training program. Answering these questions will get you on the right track:

- Can you teach the exercises and supervise them properly to ensure safety as well as proper training? If your staffing does not allow you to implement an ideal program, then don't try to. It's better to scale the program back to meet the resources available than to risk injury.
- Is lack of time a factor? If so, consider the "weight room without walls" concept, where strength training is integrated within the location and time frame of the actual practice session. This is accomplished using the natural environment, body-weight exercises, medicine balls, and stretch cords. It may seem like a compromise, but this can be very effective in sports that do not require external resistance, such as soccer, tennis, and swimming.
- What facilities and equipment are available? Do not make facilities or equipment a limiting factor in beginning a program. A few quality exercises done consistently will yield terrific results. This is especially true when beginning a program.

In designing a strength training program carefully consider the qualities of the individual athlete.

Design Rules

Now that you understand the important principles and have answered the pertinent questions about the athletes, you can start designing a program. Here are some guidelines:

Testing Strength — It is critical to test your athletes before beginning a program. When designing programs for new athletes, it is probably best to utilize projected maximums, since the 1RM can be unsafe for the inexperienced.

Time of Year — Obviously, the greatest emphasis on strength training should be during the off-season and the pre-season. But it is important to also develop a manageable program that can be continued throughout the season.

Progression — Progress from body-weight exercises to external resistance exercises both within the workout and through the training year. Also, within each workout, perform balance/stability work and core work first. Start with simple, easy-to-perform exercises, then progress to more complex movements. The key to progression is mastery. If you allow the athlete to proceed further into the program before the exercises have been mastered, there is a higher risk of injury.

Frequency — There are basically two alternatives, both of which work quite well depending on the objective. The first option is to train the entire body on alternate days three days a week. The second option uses a split routine. For example, you might train the legs and total body on Monday and Thursday and train the upper body on Tuesday and Friday.

Number of Exercises — It is best to carefully choose and limit the number of exercises. I have found that too many exercises will dilute the training effect. Determine the essential "need to do" exercises so athletes focus on the workout and not on learning new exercises.

Sets/Reps — For body-weight exercises, a range of 10 to 20 reps is necessary to force adaptation. For weight training, the traditional paradigm of sets and reps is still very valid: Use higher reps for hypertrophy development and lower reps with multiple sets for neural development.

Mode of Resistance — Depending on the objective and the phase of the program, the following resistance modes can all be used: body weight, stretch cord, medicine ball, power ball, dumbbells, and barbells. Each mode has its advantages and disadvantages depending on the specific objectives of the training program.

Duration — Generally, it is best to keep the entire strength-training session in the time range of one hour to 90 minutes. The closer to one hour, the more optimal the results.

Evaluating Results — The traditional evaluation of a strength training program has been the ability to lift more during weight training exercises or perform more repetitions on body weight exercises. In an absolute sense, that is still valid, but I think we need to go beyond that and carefully observe the carryover to the actual sport movement. While this is much more subjective, it is the ultimate goal of any strength training program. Closely observe if the athlete's ability to start and stop has improved or if there has been a reduction in injuries.

Selecting Exercises

The type of exercises you use is limited only by your imagination. However, it is important to consider the qualities of the exercises. Here are some tips:

Make Them Multi-joint — Use as many joints as possible to produce — and reduce — force.

Close the Chain — To use gravity and ground-reaction forces, choose closed-chain exercises. Whenever possible, exercises should be performed in the standing position.

Use Tri-plane Motion — Movement occurs in all three planes, sagittal, frontal, and transverse. The key to performance is movement in the transverse plane. Therefore, it is important to include rotational movement whenever possible.

Understand Amplitude — Work over the greatest range of motion that is possible to control.

Control Speed — Incorporate speed of movement that is safe and the athlete can control.

An Exercise Menu

Appropriate exercises can be selected from six categories:

1. Balance & Stability Single-Leg Squat
Perform in three positions: straight, side, and rotation — and hold each position five counts.
Balance shift: shift right, left, forward right, forward left, back right, and back left.

2. Core Exercises
Medicine ball basic rotations: tight rotation, wide rotation, over the top, figure eight, chop to ankle (stride position), and woodchop with a twist.
Medicine ball rotations and twists: standing full twist, standing half twist, half chop, and solo med-ball sit-up (both right and left).
Medicine ball wall-throw series: overhead throw, soccer throw, chest pass, standing side to side (cross in front), standing face to the wall (throw right and left, down the side), and standing back to the wall (alternate throwing right and left).
Medicine ball total-body throws: overback throw, forward through the legs, squat, and throw.

3. Lower Body
Squat & touch single-leg squat: three positions: front, side, and rotation.
Body-weight exercises: squat, lunge, and step-up.
Jump squat leg circuit: squat, lunge, and step-up.

4. Upper Body
Pulls & pushes: front pulldown, dumbbell row, incline pull-up, incline chin-up, push-up progression, rotational bench press, dumbbell bench, rhomboid, combo I (curl & press), combo II (upper cut), and arm step-up.
Stretch-cord/mini-band menu: sidestep, walk forward and back, carioca, monster walk, dynamic protraction/retraction, dynamic scarecrow, back stroke, backhand.

5. Total Body
Dumbbell high pull
Dumbbell snatch
Squat to press
Lunge & press

6. Plyometric Exercises (Jumping)
Jump rope routine
Tuck jumps
Multidirectional jumps
Ice skater
Side to side
Hops
Zig zag bound

Introductory Program

Getting Them Started

This is an introductory program for newer athletes. The theme is to emphasize body weight for two weeks. Then, starting with the third week, increase sets with each workout as the athletes progress.

Monday/Thursday:
Total Body & Legs Emphasis
Mini-band routine
Medicine ball basic rotations
Balance routine
Single-leg squat: 2 sets x 5 on each leg
Dumbbell high pull: teach on Mon
Dumbbell snatch: teach on Thurs
Body-weight squat: 2 x 10
Body-weight lunge: 10 on each leg
Body-weight step-up: 10 on each leg
Jump squat: 10
Core work: medicine ball rotations & twists

Tuesday/Friday:
Upper Body Emphasis
Mini-band routine
Medicine ball basic rotations
Balance routine
Push-up progression: regular, incline, stagger, butt up, oblique, rotation
Incline pull-up: 3 x 8
Pulldowns (front): 3 x 8
Arm step-ups: 2 x 20
Punching: 2 x 30 (15 right & 15 left)
Stretch-cord routine
Medicine ball wall throws

Work Proprioceptive Demand — The proprioceptors assist the system in generating movement in a form appropriate to the demands placed upon the system. Thus, it's important to challenge the joint and muscle receptors to provide feedback regarding joint and limb position and then reposition accordingly. This ensures that the strength will transfer to performance.

Minimize Machines — Considering the above criteria, machine training should play a minor role in strength training programs. There is a mistaken notion that it is best to begin a strength training program by using machines. Nothing could be further from the truth. Because machines provide so much stabilization, they give a false sense of security and stability that does not transfer to a free, gravitationally enriched environment. Various rowing and pulley machines are acceptable, but even those should only be a small part of the program.

Avoid Isolation Exercises — Skip all exercises that put unusual stress on one joint. They cause neural confusion because the muscle is asked to do something different in strength training than it must do in movement. Consequently, exercises like leg extensions, leg curls, concentration curls, and pec deck flys have no place in a functional strength training program. As you can see, the variables are endless. The key is to take a proactive approach by paying attention to all the factors, both big and small. Know the goals, understand the principles, and pay attention to the individual athlete and sport. Then, choose your timing and exercises consciously and carefully. ◆

A Leg To Stand On — Training the Lower Extremities

The legs are the primary source of power for sport performance, as in a great majority of sport situations they function as part of a closed kinetic chain. Without functional leg strength, an athlete cannot have speed, strength, power, or suppleness to run, jump or throw. We must think of the legs as a functional base of the whole kinetic chain. "Function is a miraculous and complex combination of systems that are linked and react with each other. In order to understand function as a whole, the parts and components of function must be appreciated." (Gray, p. 7) The leg muscles work synergistically to reduce and produce force in reaction to gravity and the ground reaction forces in the most effective manner for the required activity.

In order to strengthen the muscles of the legs, we must select exercises that meet the following functional criteria:

- The exercise should be multi-joint. If the muscle group crosses the knee and the hip, then the exercise should work at both the knee and hip. If the muscle group crosses the knee and ankle, then the exercise intended to work that muscle should work at the knee and ankle. It is preferable to select exercises that work the ankle, knee and hip together as a functional unit.
- The exercise should close the kinetic chain. The foot should be in contact with the ground supporting the body weight. This utilizes gravity and ground reaction forces. It also allows for all types of muscle action to occur in integrated tri-plane movement. In open chain work, the muscles are acting on the environment, while in closed chain work, the muscles are reacting to the environment.
- The exercise should incorporate all three planes of motion. Movement occurs in the sagittal, frontal, and transverse planes. Therefore, it is important to train the muscles to work effectively in all three planes. This means involving movements that incorporate rotational as well as side-to-side movement.
- The exercise should be over the greatest amplitude possible. Limiting the range of motion only serves to narrow the athlete's performance spectrum. The athlete should perform the exercise through the greatest range that can be controlled.
- The exercise should incorporate speed of movement, and this is relative to the exercise and the state of training or rehab. The goal is to use a rate of speed that is safe and that the athlete is able to control. Rather than limiting speed, find a rate of speed that can be controlled.
- The exercise should be of high proprioceptive demand. It should challenge the joint, muscle, and tendon receptors to provide feedback regarding joint and limb position and reposition them accordingly. The proprioceptors assist the system to generate movement in a form that it is appropriate to the demands placed upon the system. If exercises are of low proprioceptive demand, then the body will quickly adapt and not be prepared for greater demands.

The Legs are the primary source of power for most sport performance.

Typical training programs that utilize exercises like the leg extension and leg curl fail to take into account these functional criteria. These exercises may actually contribute to the problems they are designed to solve. For example, the knee extension is commonly used to strengthen the quads to help with patella femoral problems when in actuality, it increases shear force at the knee, causing even more problems. The hamstring curl is used to help prevent hamstring pulls. In fact, it may predispose the athlete to pulled hamstrings because of the imbalanced muscle development that results from doing the exercise. Programs that use these exercises are training muscles, not movements. To be functional you must train movements, not muscles. The functional goal is to prepare the legs to effectively use ground reaction forces and gravity.

The hamstring curl isolates the movement of the hamstring as a flexor at the knee. It does not bring the proximal aspect of the hamstring into play as an extensor of the hip. Various attempts have been made to make the hamstring curl more functional, including use of the standing hamstring curl, as well as emphasizing the eccentric/lowering component of the hamstring in an attempt to replicate the eccentric load that occurs in deceleration. However, changing to a standing position does not make the exercise more functional because you are still isolating the hamstring at the knee. Emphasizing the eccentric component while doing hamstring curls does not prepare the muscle for the high eccentric deceleration forces that occur when the muscle is elongated over two joints.

With the quadriceps muscle group, conventional wisdom tells us that the quad extends the knee. The primary exercise used to train this muscle group is the leg extension exercise. Functional wisdom is quite different. According to Gray, for the quads "primary closed chain function is anterior stabilization of the knee via deceleration of knee flexion" (Gray, 1994). In the mid-stance phase of the gait cycle, extension of the knee "is the result of forward momentum of the body moving over the foot and the quads' deceleration of knee flexion. Assisting with knee extension includes the muscles that decelerate the forward momentum of the tibia, including the soleus, posterior tibias, flexor hallucis longus, flexor digitorum longus, and the peroneus longus" (Gray, 1994). Functional exercise to work the quads should be closed chain exercises that cause the muscles of the lower extremity to work together synergistically. We must remember that the quads are powerful, two-joint muscles that work both at the knee and hip. Therefore, they should be trained as two-joint muscles.

Let's look at the leg curl from the point of view of conventional wisdom and then from a functional standpoint. Conventional wisdom dictates that the leg curl is an important exercise because the hamstring flexes the knee. Therefore, it is necessary to train the hamstring as a knee flexor. The primary means of accomplishing this is the leg curl exercise. Functional wisdom, on the other hand, tells us that in movement the hamstring group of muscles are two joint muscles that work at both the hip and the knee. They extend the hip and decelerate the lower leg at the knee. On foot contact, the force of gravity and ground reaction cause the knee and hip to flex, while the foot is impacting the ground. The hamstrings eccentrically decelerate hip flexion. In addition, this lengthening action stabilizes the knee in the transverse plane (with rotation). The hamstrings actually help decelerate knee flexion by slowing down forward momentum of the lower leg. (At the heel off and into the swing phase of gait, it is the eccentric force generated at the hip by the hip flexors that is transferred into hip flexion. This is what creates most of knee flexion.) Therefore, in function it is not the hamstrings that flex the knee. The mechanism of the hamstring pull injury is a great insight into hamstring function. The hamstring pulls when the hamstring muscle is elongated over two joints just as the foot hits the ground. At this point in the stride cycle, the eccentric forces are extremely high and the hamstrings are at their greatest mechanical disadvantage because the muscles are maximally stretched at the hip and the knee. This is the point when the hamstring serves a major deceleration function.

The clear choice is between joint isolation exercises and kinetic chain exercises. Joint isolation exercises create an incorrect motor program causing confusion to the muscles. If in training the muscles are asked to do one thing, then in performance, they cannot be asked to do the opposite. Kinetic chain exercises, on the other hand, work the muscles in integrated movements as part of the whole kinetic chain. In addition, for developing a training program as well as selecting exercises during rehab, the criterion is that the exercise must prevent injury as well as enhance performance. These isolated single joint leg exercises do neither. In fact, they do little to improve performance and may predispose the athlete to injury by creating incorrect motor programs and imbalanced muscular development.

What are the alternatives? All the multi-joint movements of the legs can be trained with a few very simple exercises. These drills have many variations that allow the exercises to involve more movement or be sport-specific. Conceptually, almost all movement involving the legs is reciprocal in nature; movement seldom occurs with both legs applying force together at the same time. Forces as high as three to five times body weight are not uncommon in many activities. Therefore, it is important to train the legs unilaterally when possible. Single leg movements, movements that alternate the use of the legs, or movement that is off of one leg onto the other leg offer a myriad of possibilities when selecting exercises for both rehab and conditioning.

The traditional approach for developing leg strength has been to overload the legs with heavy back squats. This approach has its advantages and disadvantages. Although the squat is the cornerstone in any functional leg strength program, it must be put into focus so that it is accomplishing the desired goal. The heavy back squat is only one method of squatting. There are several factors that must be considered when using the heavy back squat:

In selecting lower extremity exercises, function gives us a clear choice between joint isolation exercises and kinetic chain exercises.

1. Despite its common use, it is not very functional, because most sports performance occurs on one leg. The traditional squat distributes the load to both legs. It is a good exercise to develop basic leg strength and muscular hypertrophy as preparation for more specific functional work to follow, but it is not very specific.

2. It excessively loads the spine. The amount of weight necessary to overload the legs to elicit a training effect is often more weight than the spine can safely tolerate. This presents problems for the developing athlete and the older athlete.

It is important to understand that there are many variations of the squat that will make it more functional and address the previous considerations.

Performance of exercise on one leg allows a greater training effect without adding external resistance. For example, a 160-pound athlete performing an exercise on one leg will have a resistance of 160 pounds on that one leg. It allows greater speed because there is little or no external load to slow the movement, and there is better control of the proper rhythm for that exercise. It affords little stress on the spine. Single-leg work also allows for better intra-workout recovery. In other words, while one leg is working, the other leg is resting. Single-leg work allows each leg to perform the same volume of work with the same intensity. In bilateral work, it is common to see the athlete shift the load to one side or the other, which serves to further accentuate imbalances. This is especially true if there is any abnormal curvature of the spine or a significant difference in leg length. Most importantly, single-leg exercises allow extra work to be done on the weak leg in order to achieve balanced development. Balance and proprioception are optimally challenged.

How often can you work the legs? Because the legs are weight-bearing, it is not advisable to work the legs with the same frequency as the trunk and the upper extremities. It also depends on how much other activity you are doing besides leg strength work. Many weight lifters who do not do any additional exercises besides weight training movements to tax their legs do some leg work virtually every day. On the other hand, a runner or a cyclist who uses the legs extensively in their activities should probably train the legs two to three times in a seven-day cycle. If you do choose to work the legs more often, for whatever reason, it would be advisable to only use two to three exercises in a session and emphasize a particular movement. For example, one day emphasize flexion movements while the next day emphasize extension movements. However, this must be carefully correlated with the other training activities so as not to put additional stress on the legs because, as mentioned previously, the legs will not recover as quickly due to their weight bearing function in daily activity.

How about overload? How much weight should you use? Start with body weight and the force of gravity. The principle is body weight before external resistance. A note before using external resistance: Use variations that raise the proprioceptive demand. If you are in a sport that must add mass and overcome external resistance like football, or if you are a thrower in track, this principle still holds true. But be aware that you will not be able to stay with this emphasis for quite as long.

It has been my experience that when using body weight for resistance, the optimum range is 20 to 30 reps, and they must be done at a rate of one rep per second for squatting movements and as close to that rate as possible for the other movements. This adds a high-speed eccentric component, which causes residual soreness but provides a very positive training effect.

The legs are a key link in the kinetic chain. To improve performance, they must be trained functionally following the guidelines discussed in this article. ◆

References:
Gray, Gary. *Chain Reaction Plus*. Wynn Marketing, Inc. Adrian, Mich. 1994

Zhuk, V., and Martynenko, N. "An Alternative to Strength and Power Development for Young Athletes," *Modern Athlete and Coach*, Vol. 29, #3 July, 1991.

Prescription For Healthy Knees

Injuries to the anterior cruciate ligament are among the most catastrophic in sport, and there has been a lot of press about the inordinate number of these injuries among women. Although they do not occur solely in women, ACL tears are significantly more common among women than men, especially when you compare the incidence per sports participation time.

There has been a considerable amount of discussion as to why. One topic of debate is whether gender-related factors, such as monthly hormonal changes due to the menstrual cycle, contribute to the higher incidence of ACL tears in female athletes. Although more research in this area is warranted, I believe that the effects of these factors are minimal or nonexistent and to a large extent uncontrollable.

A greater factor, and one that we can control, is how we train girls and women to play sports. Not all ACL injuries are preventable — let's not get that mistaken notion — but many of them are. Contact ACL injuries are tough to prevent. The majority of non-contact ACL injuries, on the other hand, should be preventable.

Injury statistics would seem to indicate, however, that even training programs designed with an eye toward ACL injury prevention are not working. In my opinion, this is because there is too much emphasis on training methods and activities that focus on force production in a single plane, at one joint — the knee — in nonfunctional movements and positions. The emphasis, instead, needs to be on multiple-plane, multiple-joint work that puts a premium on balance and proprioception in functional positions. This is accomplished with activities that imitate the demands of the sport.

Should there be any special considerations for the female athlete? Yes, absolutely. There must be more of an emphasis placed on strength training in order to overcome the inherent difference in muscle mass between men and women. Aside from that, the exercises are the same. I will address these activities in a relatively simple program that can be implemented as part of an overall training program to not only prevent ACL injuries, but also enhance performance. And, because training equals rehab, the prevention program will have the same look and feel as a functional rehab program and can be used equally well in either setting. But first, in order to understand how to prevent ACL injuries, we must understand the mechanism of the injury.

From Cause To Prevention

Generally, ACL tears result from a valgus load with external rotation of the tibia on the femur while the foot is fixed on the ground. According to Mary Lloyd Ireland, MD, of the Kentucky Sports Medicine Center, in Lexington, KY, and her colleagues, the "inability to decelerate the hip, knee, or ankle in all planes of motion is a major factor in ACL tears"(Ireland, et al., p 101). She and her coauthors go on to address the noncontact nature of most ACL injures:

> ". . . noncontact injuries almost always occur during deceleration of the body. These occur when the athlete lands from a jump, decelerates during the sudden lowering before initiating acceleration into the jump, or decelerates on the plant leg prior to a cutting motion. Deceleration needs to occur quickly, through a relatively small excursion of joint motion, and in the transverse, sagittal, and frontal planes of motion. The knee is influenced by the lack of control and stability from forces above and below. The excessive strain and rate of strain play a prominent part in ACL failure" (Ireland, et al., p. 104).

If these are the causes, then this is where we need to look for the solution. We must design a prevention program that puts a premium on the ability to control the gravitational loads and ground-reaction forces that occur in deceleration.

Preventing ACL injuries starts with taking the focus off the knees and shifting training to the entire kinetic chain.

In order to do this, we must shift our thinking away from traditional exercises and training methods that emphasize force production to a more balanced program involving force reduction and proprioception. In other words, we must get beyond quad strengthening using single-joint exercises like the leg extension and hamstring strengthening that uses a leg-curl apparatus. Instead, we must train in a weight-bearing position in order to better utilize the forces of gravity and ground reaction and to fully activate the appropriate proprioceptive feedback mechanisms in the joints, ligaments, tendons, and muscles. The emphasis needs to be on training integrated movement, not isolated muscles.

This information is certainly not new or revolutionary. Yet, we are still paying too much attention to the knee in isolation and not enough attention to the knee as a link in the kinetic chain. According to Gary Gray, PT, a leader in the field of functional training, "The knee is stuck in the middle with no place to go and few places to hide." It is often a helpless victim of what is happening at the joints above and below. When constructing an effective ACL injury prevention program, the focus needs to shift to the hip above and the foot/ankle below the knee. Following are some other critical points to consider:

Multi-joint Focus — In order to produce force, we use as many joints as possible, but we tend to forget that we need to use the corresponding number of joints to reduce force. We do not jump just by extending at the knee; we use triple extension of the ankle, knee, and hip. Therefore, in landing, we must bend all three joints to absorb shock and reduce force. The knee, by itself, is not designed to withstand the forces that are imposed upon it in athletic activities like landing from a jump or cutting at full speed. We could work on the knee and the muscles that surround the knee forever and never really rectify the ACL problem.

Joint Awareness — Another aspect of the equation that has been completely ignored in prevention and training is consideration for proprioception, or joint position sense, which is based on feedback from receptors in the joint, ligaments, tendons, and muscles. This, coupled with kinesthesia—the sensation of joint motion and acceleration—must be a key consideration in each exercise. It is these components that lend quality and control to the movements.

Replicate Gait — Careful consideration must be given to the selection of the exercises and their actual performance. Unilateral work on one leg and reciprocal work on alternating legs is preferable to work done in a bilateral stance with both feet on the ground. Look at the gait cycle and the demands of actual athletic performance: seldom is work done with both feet in contact with the ground. Most often, movement involves shifting from one foot to the other. That is not to say that no work will be done in a bilateral stance. Rather, it is a matter of emphasis.

Stability vs. Flexibility — Where does flexibility enter into the equation? Joint stability is a much more important factor than joint mobility. It is best to think of Gary Gray's concept of "mostability," which is the correct amount of motion in the correct plane at the correct time at the correct joint. With this in mind, hip mobility is of paramount importance. At the knee and ankle, stability is most important. The emphasis should be on as large a range as the athlete can control. The key is control.

Progressing To Control — Motor control, coupled with proper strengthening, is the cornerstone of a prevention program. This must be combined with dynamic core stability work in order to maintain proper pelvic alignment. This core stability work must be done in functional positions in order to be effective.

Neuromuscular control is influenced by proprioceptive information based on collective kinesthetic, vestibular, and visual information. Because of the nature and quality of input from these sensory systems, all of these components must be incorporated into a prevention/training program. These components can be sequentially added as part of a progression. The steps in a sound progression are:

Easy-to-hard — Begin with exercises that the athlete can easily do and then progress to more difficult exercises.

Simple-to-complex — Start with simple movements, then add complexity as the athlete masters these.

Known-to-unknown — Begin with exercises that occur in an environment the athlete is familiar with, then go to unknown areas that challenge the athlete's proprioceptive and kinesthetic systems.

Stable-to-unstable — Start with exercises in a stable, controlled environment and gradually add instability and a less-controlled environment, which challenge the proprioceptive and kinesthetic senses to the maximum. Progress in the following sequence: barefoot > airex pad > half foam roller > Dyna Disc > reaction to visual, auditory, or kinesthetic stimuli. The progression must be criteria-based. This means that the first step must be mastered before proceeding to the next step. The criteria are quality of movement, control through a full range of movement and speed of movement with control.

The Prevention Program: LEPPP™

I developed LEPPP™ (the Lower Extremity Prevention and Performance Program™) with input from scores of other performance coaches over the last 30 years to help address these types of injuries. The following exercises are presented in sequence according to degree of difficulty. They are best done as an extension of the warm up at the start of a practice or strength training session. They also can be an effective homework assignment for athletes who have a particular problem area that must be addressed. The key to the success of this program is how it is put together and sequenced. This requires an evaluation of the demands of the athlete's particular sport the athlete's position within that sport and most importantly, the qualities of each individual athlete. This is highly individual. Carefully pick exercises from each category, and adjust sets and reps from the general guidelines given to fit the needs of your athletes.

Mobility

The emphasis here is on dynamic movements through a large range of motion with control.

Hurdle Walks
Set up low hurdles spaced just far enough to allow the athlete to plant one foot before having to walk over (or under) the next hurdle, alternating the lead foot with each hurdle.
• Over the top
• Over and under

Leg Swings
• Flexion/extension
• Abduction/adduction

Mini-Band Routine
With a large rubber band around his or her ankles, have the athlete do the following:

- Side step
- Walking: forward and backward
- Carioca
- Monster walk (have the athlete walk while maintaining a squat position. This forces him or her to rotate his or her lead leg outward and forward, working several muscle groups at once)

Balance and Proprioception

Single-Leg Squat Balance
The athlete should start standing on one leg, squat down to a position just above a half-squat position. The position of the free (nonsupporting) leg will determine the dominant plane.
- Sagittal: Free leg straight ahead
- Frontal: Free leg extended out to the side
- Transverse: Free leg rotated back

Hold the squat position for 10 seconds. One set in each position is recommended.

Balance Shift
Start from a basic athletic position. Hold each position for 10 seconds. Again, one set is recommended.
- Shift onto left foot
- Shift onto right foot
- Step forward onto left foot
- Step forward onto right foot
- Step backward onto left foot
- Step backward onto right foot

Balance Board
Have the athlete start out with both feet on the balance board and then progress to such things as balancing with eyes closed and balancing while catching a ball. Then, possibly have him or her repeat the progression on one foot.

BOSU™
Single-leg squat balance (10-second hold). Repeat same as before, but now change the proprioceptive demand by adding the unstable surface.
- Sagittal
- Frontal
- Transverse

Strength (High Force)

The emphasis here is on bodyweight exercises using gravitational loading based on the principle of bodyweight before external resistance.

Squat and Touch
The athlete should stand on one leg with the foot of the other just above the ankle of the supporting leg. The hand on the side of the supporting leg should be on the hip. The athlete will squat down bending at the ankle, knee, and hip while reaching down and touching predetermined spots on the ground (left, left/front, front, right/front, right, right/back, and left/back) with the hand on the free-leg side. He or she should repeat with the other leg. Have him or her do each leg two to four times.

Squat and Touch and Reach
The same as the previous exercise, but after squatting and touching, the athlete should reach up as high as possible.

Single-Leg Squat
Have the athlete start standing on one leg, then squat down by proportionally bending ankle, knee, and hip to a half-squat position. The position of the free (non-supporting) leg will determine the dominant plane.
- Sagittal
- Frontal
- Transverse

Single-Leg Squat and Catch (3-Kg Medicine Ball)
The athlete should start standing on one leg, squat down by proportionally bending ankle, knee, and hip to a half-squat position. Then, he or she will pick up a medicine ball, which is placed approximately six inches in front of the supporting foot. Have him or her throw the medicine ball up to just above head height, then catch the ball and return it to the starting position while squatting down.

Rotational Lunge
Have the athlete rotate back and to the side while performing a lunge (stepping back at about a 45-degree angle). He or she should immediately return to the starting position.

Rotational Lunge with a Catch (3-Kg Medicine Ball) Same as the previous exercise but have a partner throw a ball as the athlete is lunging back.

Plyometric (High Speed/High Force)

Multidirectional Jumps/Hops
The athlete jumps (two-foot landings) or hops (one-foot landings) forward/side, right/side, left/backward.

Rotational Bounds
The athlete should step back and to the side and immediately rebound back to the starting position. Then, have him or her execute the same movement to the other side. He or she should continue to alternate for the prescribed number of repetitions.

Lateral Restart Jumps
Have the athlete execute two consecutive jumps sideways and then one jump back in the opposite direction. He or she should repeat this pattern of jumps five times.

BOSU™
Jump, jump, stick (start on two feet and land on two feet). Hop, hop, stick (start on one foot and land on one foot).

Movement / Motor Control

Retro Running
Have the athlete run backwards for up to about 30 yards.
- Level
- Uphill

ABC™/ Agility Ladder™

The athlete should perform the lateral movements with a focus on getting the feet back down to the ground quickly. ◆

References

Ireland, Mary Lloyd, Gaudette, and Cook, Scoot. *ACL Injuries in the Female Athlete*, Journal of Sport Rehabilitation, vol. 6, 1997, pp. 97-110.

Perrin, David H. *Anterior Cruciate Ligament Injury in the Female Athlete*, Journal of Athletic Training, vol. 34 no. 2, April-June 1999.

The Road To France — World Cup 1998

Beginning in September 1995, I had the opportunity to work with Roy Wegerle. Roy was a member of the 1994 US World Cup soccer team where he saw limited playing time due to rehabilitation from knee surgery. The following year he returned to play in England, where he reinjured the same knee. In September 1995, he was introduced to me by Ken Shields, his former trainer with the Tampa Bay Rowdies of the old NASL. Ken felt that I would be able to help Roy with a functional rehab program and a return to play program. We were able to work on a program for several weeks before he had to attend a National Team training camp. We knew that there was not enough time to get back to 100%, but it was a start. Due to his inability to perform consistently, he was dropped from the national team. There was also pressure to play due to the beginning of the inaugural MLS season where Roy was one of the allocated players to the Colorado Rapids. He was able to play the 1996 MLS season, despite missing most of training camp with recurrent problems with the knee after his eighth knee surgery. He was never 100% at any time during the 1996 season.

In the middle of the 1997 season, Roy was traded to DC United where he was instrumental in helping them to their second straight MLS championship. Possibly because his playing time was limited in Colorado, his knee began to feel better, and he was able to begin a more consistent strength training regimen. In October of 1997, he was added to the National Team where he played a key role in the US qualifying for the 1998 World Cup. Despite this success, he felt he was still not 100%. Due to a break in the schedule, he had two months off without having any team commitments and was able to focus completely on training. In this article, I will detail the goals, objectives, and implementation of Roy's program in preparation for the 1998 World Cup.

Roy approached his training with a mission and a sense of purpose that I have seldom seen in my years of coaching. He knew what he had to do and how to push himself, which was a key. As is typical for most world class athletes in both team and individual sports, there are seldom any lengthy breaks from competition where they can properly train, rehabilitate, and generally recharge the batteries. The period of time from the last World Cup qualifying game in November until the start of National Team training camp in January afforded Roy this unique opportunity.

Even though this program was designed for a world class athlete, the principles are applicable to players at all levels. One important factor is that Roy's soccer skills were well developed after years of play, so that skill reacquisition was a minimal consideration and the focus could be entirely on physical preparation.

Roy's progress to the World Cup is an application of the axiom that: rehab = training and training = rehab.

The objectives of the program were:

- *Injury Rehabilitation* — Because the rehab process never had been completed, this had to be the first objective and was the focus for the first two weeks of the program. It actually never ceased to be an emphasis, but the focus shifted to a prehabilitation emphasis in order to fit into the normal training program. The elements of rehab were constantly threaded throughout the program.
- *Performance Enhancement* — Once the rehab and prehab were thoroughly addressed, the remainder of the program focused on what needed to be done to help him improve as a player. Particular attention was given to speed, lateral speed and agility, and specific strength in order to take full advantage of his soccer skills.
- *Confidence Building* — This was a big part of the whole program. He needed to feel completely secure in planting, cutting, and shooting off the "weak" leg. Everything was designed to progressively increase the stress and simulate every possible movement and situation that could occur in a game.
- *Education* — Learn how to continue his training within the context of training camp and the season by establishing a routine of training. This routine had to be practical and efficient.

To accomplish these objectives, it was necessary to emphasize the following concepts:

Warm up to play. Don't play to warm up. A thorough and complete active warm-up was done at the start of each session. The warm-up was specific to the objective of the session. If the session called for a straight ahead speed emphasis, then the warm-up was tailored to meet that objective.

Condition to kick and run. Don't kick and run to condition. This was accomplished by breaking the components of soccer skill into the fundamental movements and then strengthening in the specific ranges of those movements.

Condition and prepare the whole body using the kinetic chain concept. The body is a link system with all parts working together to produce efficient movement. Failure to understand and use these concepts has the negative effect of predisposing the player to injury as well as improper skill development. Soccer is looked upon as a lower body sport, but without a strong core all the lower body work is for naught. Therefore, a large amount of work was devoted to dynamic core stabilization activities.

Roy's specific soccer conditioning program was based on the application of the following principles:
- Dynamic postural alignment and muscular balance are the basis for all training. Posture is a dynamic quality that involves movement and the ability to handle a variety of positions.
- Fundamental movement skill must be mastered and continually reinforced before specific sport skill. The fundamental movement skills consist of four broad categories: locomotor skills, nonlocomotor skills, manipulative skills, and movement awareness. These fundamental movement skills are the basis for more complex soccer specific movements. Soccer specific movements are composed of a series of linked fundamental movement skills. If the player has a rich repertoire of motor skills to draw from, not only is it is easier to acquire soccer skill, but the athlete is less prone to injury.
- Body weight before external resistance. The game of soccer does not require the ability to move an opponent or to overcome large external resistance. Therefore, the strength training emphasized bodyweight exercises augmented by a weight vest for resistance.
- Structural (core) strength before extremity strength. Strength through the core was an ancillary objective of each exercise. All movement starts from the stronger, slower muscles surrounding the athletes center of gravity and moves out to the extremities. The core acts as a force couple which connects the upper body to the lower extremities. A weak core will cause improper postural alignment, which will detract from correct skill and predispose the player to injury. The main methods of working the core in a functional manner as it relates to soccer is through medicine ball training.
- Joint integrity before joint mobility. This was accomplished by selecting exercises that stressed multi-joint as well as multi-plane movements that were high in proprioceptive demand.

The program was based on the five step sport development model.

Step #1 — The Sport: Soccer

It is important to condition for the demands of the game of soccer. Soccer requires quick starts and quick stops. There is a constant interplay of force production and force reduction with most injuries occurring during the force reduction phase of stopping and kicking. Roy plays forward, which demands speed, game awareness, and the ability to stop quickly and change direction. Consequently, the emphasis was on speed and power production. Less than 2% of the total distance covered by a player during a match is with the ball. Each match requires 1,000 to 1,200 bouts of action that require quick changes of direction, as well as precise execution of game skills. Sprints average about 15 meters and generally occur about once every 90 seconds. There are numerous jumps to win balls in the air.

Step #2 — The Athlete

What physical qualities did Roy possess relative to the demands of soccer and his position? He was evaluated relative to the following parameters:

Work Capacity — His work capacity was high. The cumulative effect of years of training enabled him to tolerate a high workload and recover.

Strength/Power — He had great relative strength; he could handle his own bodyweight well.

Speed — This quality needed work because it had been compromised by the down time from injury, which limited his ability to work on speed. Roy did have above average speed and outstanding ability to accelerate. This needed to be emphasized so he could regain those qualities.

Coordination and Skill — This was outstanding. He had great body awareness, which enhanced the reacquisition of movements.

Dynamic Flexibility — This needed emphasis. The emphasis here was on mostability so that he could control the necessary ranges of motion.

Body Composition — This was not an issue; he was very lean.

Step #3 — The System

Everything had to be Manageable, that is it needed to be accomplished given the facilities, equipment, and personnel available. The results had to be Measurable in order to be quantified. They needed to be Motivational so Roy could see the reason for the training and relate it to his improvement as a player.

There was no single joint work. Everything was functional based on the simplest component, which is the gait cycle: all movement in soccer is off one leg onto the other. Speed of movement was the first consideration in the functional strength training exercises because he had to be able to handle high speed eccentric loading as demanded by the game. The next step was to increase the amplitude of the movement and then add reaction. Everything was worked in a proprioceptively demanding environment. The training components that made up the system were:

    Speed
        Straight Ahead Speed (SAS)
        Lateral Speed & Agility (LSA)
    Strength/Power
        Body Weight Exercises
        Medicine Ball Work
        Plyometrics
    Stamina
        Speed Endurance
    Suppleness
        Mostability
    Skill

Philosophically, facilities or equipment would not be a limiting factor. Therefore, in the last two weeks of the program, most everything was done on the field.

Step #4 — The Plan

In preparing the training plan, I considered the following questions: Where were we starting? Where were we going? How could the program be implemented? What roadblocks would occur along the way? To prepare for the length of the competitive season, it was necessary to design a practical periodization plan for the time available. The emphasis was on timing of the application of training components. The fundamental cycle was a work to recovery ratio of 3:1 shifting to 2:1 in the last two weeks before training camp. A detailed long term plan was not feasible because too many of the factors would be out of Roy's or my control as he progressed into the MLS season. A key component was active rest and regeneration in the form of pool work and massage.

Step #5 — The Evaluation

In this case, the evaluation was based on careful observation of the drills within training rather than a formal test battery. Testing = Training and Training = Testing, so that each session was a test to provide feedback as to the effectiveness of that session, as well as where to go with the next session. Careful observation of game and practice performance was also very important. We knew that when he reported to National Team Camp in January, there would be formal evaluation in the form of field tests. Some of the training was directed toward performance on these tests to establish his position on the team. The National Team tests were:

- Vertical Jump
- Agility Test
- 300 Shuttle Test
- Flying start 40 yard Sprint
- "Beep Test"

He performed very well on these tests, which served as a positive springboard into the training camp.

Training Program

Wednesday, December 10, 1997
Warm-up
    15 Minutes on Treadmill
    Mini Band Routine
Remedial Work
    Med Ball Moving Catches
    Med Ball Wall Throws—Throw & Catch on One Leg
    Med Ball Partner Balance Throws on Half Foam Roller
    Retro Hill Runs x 6 @ 75 yards
Strength Training
    Retro Step-up
    Step Downs - a) Anterior b) Lateral b) Posterior
    Bodyweight Squat & Press Overhead with Med Ball
    Bodyweight Squat & Reach Out with Med Ball
    Single Leg Squat & Press Overhead with Med Ball
    Single Leg Squat & Reach Out with Med Ball
    Diagonal Lunge
    Lunge & Reach
Cooldown
    Partner Stretch
    Physioball Routine

Thursday, December 11, 1997
Warm-up
    Bike 10 Minutes
    Mini Band Routine
Remedial Work
    Med Ball Moving Catches
    Med Ball Wall Throws - Throw & Catch on One Leg
    Med Ball Partner Balance Throws on Half Foam Roller

Thursday, December 11, 1997 (continued...)
    Retro Hill runs x 6 @ 75 yards
    Leaning Tower
    Step Downs with Reaction Coach™
Agility
    Dot Drill
    Low Box Quickstep
        a) Straight Ahead b) Lateral
Strength Training
    Bodyweight Squat & Press Overhead with Med Ball
        (Add Weight Vest)
    Bodyweight Squat & Reach Out with Med Ball
        (Add Weight Vest)
    Single Leg Squat & Press Overhead with Med Ball
    Single Leg Squat & Reach Out with Med Ball
    Multi Plane Cobra Lunge
    Lateral Bound & Stick - Hold 5 Count
    Leg Circuit x 2 or 3 with 1 Minute Recovery
        Between Circuits
    (Follow circuit with balance on Med Ball for stability)
    Pushup routine x 2 sets
Cooldown
    Static Stretch
    Physioball Routine

Friday, December 12, 1997
Recovery/Regeneration
    Pool Session Emphasis on Large Ranges of Movement
    Massage

Saturday, December 13, 1997
Rest

Summary

The success of the program was directly related to Roy's hard work and constant input. This was a program designed specifically for Roy based on systematic sound training principles. In this article, I have emphasized the principles and thought processes that went into formulating the program, rather than specific workouts.

At the conclusion of the January training camp, Roy scored the winning goal in a match against Sweden and was named MVP of the game. That was another positive step on the road to France. ◆

Round 'n' Round — Circuit Training

What is Circuit Training?

Circuit training is essentially interval strength training. It consists of a series of strength training as well as general fitness exercises where the athlete moves from station to station in a predetermined sequence. While at a particular station, the exercise is either performed for a set amount of time or a predetermined number of repetitions. The athlete then proceeds immediately to the next exercise and either immediately begins the next exercise or takes a prescribed rest before beginning the next exercise. Circuit training is a very effective method to raise work capacity levels, target specific areas of the body or physical qualities, change body composition, and develop strength endurance. In a team or a group setting, it will enable a large number of athletes to safely train at one time.

Circuit training is certainly not new, although it has recently been rediscovered by the general fitness population. Morgan and Adamson, in Great Britain, are generally credited as the people who systematized the approach in the fifties. It has traditionally been used as a means of building work capacity in preparation for strength training programs. Typically it has been utilized at the start of a strength training program. I believe that is too narrow a use. It is a very versatile training method that can be utilized throughout the training year. It is also appropriate for use in rehabilitation. Just as with any training method, it is important to know the theory and methodological basis before actually utilizing the method.

I have found it useful to divide circuit training into six categories (see sample circuits) based on their specific training objective:

Basic Circuits — Usually utilizing bodyweight or minimal external resistance. Seldom more than twelve exercises. Very basic in their design and application. No complex movements.

Fitness Circuits — As the name implies, the specific goal here is to raise general fitness levels and reduce body fat. The circuits are longer in duration and more complex in construction. Usually an aerobic component is included.

Biased Circuits — Circuits designed to place emphasis on one particular area of the body. These circuits are usually rep-based and relatively simple in construction.

Advanced Circuits — More complex construction involving more exercises.

Weight Lifting Complexes — Combination of three to six weight training and Olympic lifting movements utilized as a stand alone session or a preparatory activity for a specific strength training workout to follow.

Power Endurance Circuits — Jumping or medicine ball exercises done in a circuit format designed to simulate the power demands of sports that require high power production but still induce a fatigued state.

Circuit Training-Goals

- Develop strength endurance, which is the capacity to express strength in a climate of fatigue.
- Increase work capacity, which is the overall ability to tolerate a workload and recover from that workload.
- Enable large numbers to train at one time. This is particularly useful with teams or when training time available is limited.
- Target specific areas to bias the circuit to train a particular area of the body in order to prepare for heavier work to follow.

Basic Principle

Circuit Training is the primary method for the development of strength and power endurance.

Strength before strength endurance. Master the exercises first which is neural adaptation. Through neural adaptation, the athlete will show significant gains. Neural adaptations occur in as short a time as fourteen to twenty-one days. Also, make sure that you can do the exercise with correct technique and rhythm before adding an endurance component. Following this principle will lessen the risk of injury and insure better long term training adaptations. Traditionally, circuit programs have been the first phase in a strength training program. This is not advisable because the athlete does not yet have the strength to endure.

Circuit Training — Construction Guidelines

- The exercises must be tailored to meet individual needs and rates of improvement. One size does not fit all. A fitness circuit for a 400 meter runner should be different than a circuit for a basketball team.
- The exercise must be strenuous. Remember the one goal is to raise work capacity. If the exercises are too easy, there will be little or no adaptive response.
- The exercises must be simple, since skill will breakdown when fatigued. If complex exercises are used, put them early in the circuit where the effect of fatigue will be minimized.
- The exercises must be standardized in order for the athlete to know what he or she is doing and measure progress. This allows for comparison in order to gauge progress.
- Understand the bias or alternate body parts and movements. By sequencing exercises in a certain manner or the selection of exercises, it is possible to bias the circuit to a particular body part.

Circuit Training — Criteria

Time — A certain exercise for a specified period of time or a total time for the complete circuit. Even with time as a criteria it is advisable to count the number of repetitions performed during that period.

Rest/Recovery — The rest between exercises and

between trips through the circuit. Circuits can also be done continuously without rest. They can also be constructed so that there are periods with rest and series of exercises without rest. For example, a 30 exercise circuit could be constructed in the following manner: 10 exercises could be performed for 30 seconds with 15 seconds rest; the next 10 exercises could be done with no rest; the next 10 exercises could be done for 30 seconds with 15 seconds rest.

Reps — How many times you execute each exercise. Test for maximum number of reps and then perform a certain percentage of max reps or a set number of reps which could be determined arbitrarily.

Trips — Number of times through the circuit. One time through the circuit is considered one trip. The circuit can be constructed so that there is rest between trips or the circuit can be done continuously.

Load — The amount of resistance the athlete uses, either external loading or body weight.

Progression

Start simple with basic exercises that utilize the minimum of bodyweight and equipment following the principle of body weight before external resistance. Once the athlete can handle bodyweight circuit with a degree of proficiency, then add more complex movements. The next step would be to add equipment or implements that offer external resistance.

Record Keeping

Based on the criteria of the respective circuit, it is important to keep track of the athletes' progress. One method is to pair off the athletes so that one works and one records during their rest period. If a recorder is available, have the athlete call out reps to a recorder during the rest phase or have the athlete self record.

Administration

Set up the circuit so that that there is adequate space to execute the exercises as well as to move between stations. Give careful attention to the flow of traffic for safety and ease of coaching. For time based circuits, it is helpful to have a circuit timer that sounds a loud audible sound at the beginning and end of each work and rest period.

Sample Circuits

The following are sample circuits from each category. They are actual circuits that I have used in training athletes.

Basic Circuits

Basic Circuit — Use this with a novice athlete or at the start of the training year. I have used this with track athletes in the first two weeks of a preparation phase and then have added exercises as their fitness levels improved.
Criteria: The circuit is rep based but it is also helpful to keep track of the total time of the circuit.
    Push-up x 10
    Three-Position Sit-up x 10
    Body Weight Squat x 10
    Mountain Climber x 20 each leg
    Cross Crawl x 10
    Squat Thrust x 10

Med Ball Circuit — This is a circuit that I especially like to use with throwers, tennis players, and swimmers.
Criteria: The circuit is rep based.
    Overhead Throw x 20
    Soccer Throw x 20
    Chest Pass x 20
    Side Throw 10 each side
    Cross In Front x 10 each side
    Around the Back x 10 each side

Biased Circuits

Leg Circuit—This is a circuit that I have in virtually every sport. It is terrific work to lay a foundation for the specific work to follow.
Criteria: The circuit is rep based.
    Body Weight Squat x 20
    Body Weight Lunge x 20
    Body Weight Step-up x 20
    Jump Squat x 10

Fitness Circuits

Slide Board/Core Circuit — A good circuit to use in rehabilitation of athletes coming off of lower extremity injuries. It is low impact but very demanding.
Criteria: The circuit is time based.
30 second work - 15 second recovery
Trips: Two four trips, no rest between trips.
Alternate Russian Twist, Sit-up, LA Sit-up, Diagonal Chop & Wood Chop with slide board.

Burn With Vern Circuit — This is a good circuit to use if someone has to lose body fat and raise overall work capacity. Even though I am not a fan of crash programs, you can see quick results with this.
The circuit is constructed so that there is an upper body exercise, followed by a core exercise, followed by a lower body exercise. (See Table One)

Field/Court Circuits

Criteria: The circuit is rep and time based.
I have used this type of circuit with basketball players and tennis players at the end of the off season phase as a transition into more specific conditioning work.
Reps: Each station has a prescribed number of repetitions. Between each exercise, there is a prescribed activity that is done for a set distance where the next exercise is performed.
Trips: Begin with one trip through the circuit and work up to five trips through the circuit with three minutes rest between circuits.

    Push-up x 20
    Sidestep
    Med Ball Sit-up x 10
    Carioca

Body Weight Squat x 20
  Run
Med Ball Chest Pass x 20
  Crossover Run
Med Ball Chops x 10 each side
  Skipping
Lunge x 10 each leg
  Run

Advanced Circuits

Dumbbell Matrix — I use this with soccer players and other athletes who do not need to bulk up, but require strength in all planes of motion. This is a circuit developed in conjunction with Gary Gray to address all planes of movement.

Criteria: The circuit is rep based.
Reps: Each exercise is three repetitions
Trips: Perform all sagittal plane exercises, then all frontal plane exercises, then all transverse plane exercises. That is one trip. The goal is three trips.

Sagittal (S) Frontal (P) Transverse (T)
Legs
  (S1) Anterior Lunge
  (F1) Side Lunge
  (T1) Posterior Lunge

Trunk
  (S2) High Pull
  (F2) Dynamic Side Bend
  (T2) One Arm Rotational Snatch

Upper
  (S3) Alternate Db Press
  (F3) Lateral Step & Raise
  (T3) V Across

Power Endurance Circuit

Jump Circuit—Use with soccer, basketball, and 400 meter runners. Anyone that has to express power in a climate of fatigue.
Use lower amplitude, less technically demanding exercises.
Criteria: The circuit is rep based.
Trips: Two to three trips.
  Ankle Bounce x 30
  Side To Side x 20
  Scissors Jump x 20
  Ice Skater x 10 each side
  Jump Squat x 10

Recommended Resources

Hartmann, Jurgen and Tunneman, Harold, *Fitness and Strength Training*, Berlin: Sportverlag, 1989.

Scholich, Manfred, *Circuit Training*, Berlin: Sportverlag 1986.

Ward, Paul E. and Ward, Robert D., *The Encyclopedia Of Weight Training: Weight Training For General Conditioning, Sport And Body Building*, Laguna Hills, California: QPT Publications, 1997.

Table 1: Burn with Vern Circuit

Upper-Body Exercise	Core Exercise	Lower-Body Exercise
Push-up	Med Ball Standing Twist	Bodyweight Squat
Curl + Press	Standing Twist	Lunge
Reverse Curl + Inward Press	Diagonal Chops	Step-up
Incline Press	Rhomboid	Ice Skater
Body Blade	Alternate DB Press	High Step-up
Curls	Pyramid Push-up	Overhead Squat
Med Ball Overhead Throw	Front Pulldown	Lateral Step-up
Med Ball Chest Pass Arm Step-ups	Reverse-Grip Front Pulldown	Crossover Single-Leg Squat
Crunch	Med NBall Two-Position Sit-up	Low Box Stepover
	Rotational Push-up	Squat Thrust

Each exercise is done for a prescribed amount of time.

Monday
30 seconds work
15 seconds rest
regular circuit

Wednesday
45 seconds work
15 seconds rest
60 seconds aerobic work after every three exercises

Friday
45 seconds work
15 seconds rest
45 seconds aerobic work after each exercise

More Power To You

The quest to develop power as a means of improving sports performance is never-ending. Training methods run the gamut from heavy weight training, to light, fast weight training, to plyometrics where the acceleration and deceleration of the body is the overload. While all of these methods produce results, the problem is that the results are not always commensurate with the training time invested.

As a coach, I have tried many different methods with varying degrees of success and have always felt that there should be a more systematic way to approach power development. My continuing search has led me to the work of Australian sport scientists, Greg Wilson and Robert Newton, whose research appeals to me because of its practical application. In this article, I will attempt to summarize their findings and give some practical ideas on the implementation of their concepts.

Strength and Speed

Power is the application of strength combined with speed. Strength is only concerned with the application of force; it is expressed by the formula F x D (where F = force and D = distance), thus the time of the application of force is of no consideration. Power is expressed by the formula F x D/Time. Therefore, in exhibiting power, speed is of the essence. Power is the quality needed for performance in the athletic arena, where most movements take place in less than .3 of a second.

The training methods to achieve this kind of power are not new and primarily involve ballistic work. Examples are best found in track and field, where these methods have been used for years by jumpers and throwers (and more recently by sprinters and hurdlers) because this arena demands the highest expression of explosive power to propel a body or an implement with maximal velocity.

Rethinking Weightlifting

High power production is best represented in such sport activities as the shot put, throwing a baseball, or swinging a golf club. The common characteristic of all these activities is that the implement or ball is accelerated progressively throughout the movement until release or contact occurs.

When we use traditional weight training to achieve high power production, we run into one large limitation: progressive acceleration is curtailed. As mentioned above, to achieve maximal power, the body or body part holding the bar or the implement must accelerate throughout the movement. However, to safely weight train, the bar must achieve zero velocity at the end of the concentric phase of the movement. In other words, near the end of an exercise, whether it is a squat, clean, or bench press, the bar must slow down in preparation for stopping.

Research has shown that in a maximal lift, 23 percent of the movement accounts for deceleration of the bar. In a lift at 81 percent of maximum, the deceleration phase accounts for 52 percent of the concentric movement. This is one of the major limitations of weight training for the development of maximal power.

In the search to utilize weights to raise explosive power, one method that has been advocated is to lift lighter weights quickly. Superficially, it appears that the bar is moving fast, but even this approach does not solve the problem as the bar is accelerated for only a small time at the first part of the movement. The rest of the lift produces very little force since the work is directed at slowing down and stopping the bar at the end of the movement.

In addition to the deceleration problem, traditional weight training is unable to imitate specific sport movements. This is true of both machines and free weights. Therefore, traditional weightlifting is not functional in developing sport-specific power.

That is not to say that weight training is unimportant. Much to the contrary, it is very important to have a base of absolute strength, which weight training can provide. However, it must be used at the proper place as part of an overall program instead of being the sole focus of the program.

Achieving Power Training

So how do we achieve Maximal Power Training (MPT)? According to Wilson, "Maximal explosive power training involves performance of dynamic weight training at the load which maximizes mechanical power output." This involves lifting loads in the range of 30 to 45 percent of maximum at high speed.

Based on the previous discussion, it should be obvious that the exercises must not be typical weight-training exercises where the bar reaches zero velocity at the end of the movement. This would be counterproductive to the stated goal of raising explosive power.

One solution is to think of MPT as a marriage between strength training and plyometrics. "Maximal power training could be considered a form of plyometric training that is specifically performed at a load which

Achieving sport-specific, explosive power through weight training continues to confound coaches. Here are some new ideas on the topic.

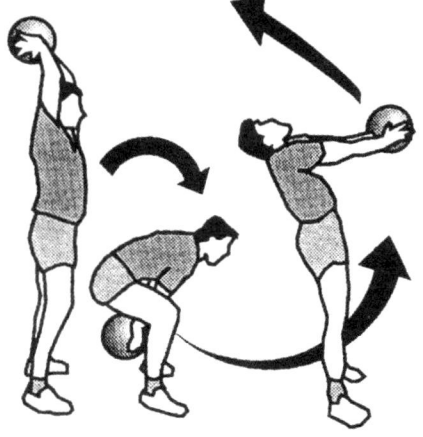

Figure One: Medicine Ball Triple Extension Throw Backward

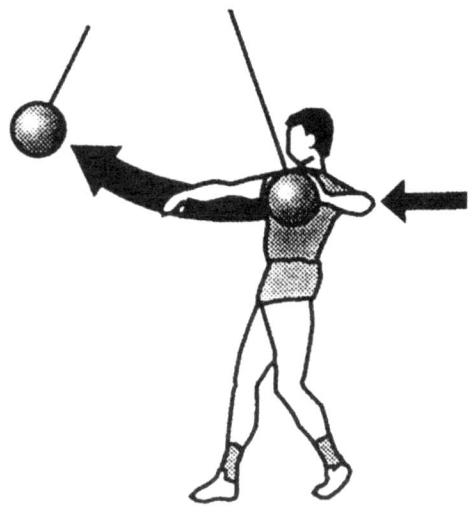

Figure Two: Pendulum Swing

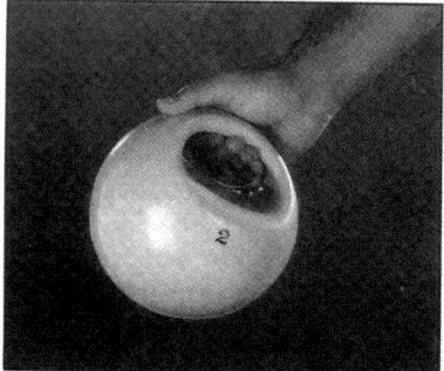

Figure Three: Power Ball

maximizes the power output of the exercise." The loading is greater than plyometrics because more resistance than body weight is used, but lighter than traditional weight training.

In selecting exercises for maximal power training, the key is to find those that allow for the production of the highest possible force throughout the entire range of motion. One of the best examples of this is the weighted squat jump. According to Baker, "The multiple repetition jump squats are associated with power outputs usually only generated by elite weightlifters during the second pull of the jerk thrust." He goes on to conclude, " ... multiple repetition jump squats may provide an excellent alternative or supplement to the traditional Olympic weightlifting style movements for the development of speed-strength."

Incorporating these methods of MPT is not without hazards, however. The danger is that, due to external loading, the exercises have greater impact forces as well as greater contact times at a slower velocity than plyometric training, where there is no external load. This makes it imperative that athletes have a very good training base or they will be at greater risk of injury.

In addition, using MPT involves a paradigm shift for athletes who have relied almost exclusively on heavy external loading through weight training. It also demands more imagination and creativity on the part of the coach to develop programs that serve the needs of the individual athletes relative to the power demands of their sport.

Sample Exercises

Plyo Power System — This is an exercise that Wilson and Newton used for their research. It involves a modified Smith machine with a computer-controlled braking device to catch the bar after it is released. It is the safest way to incorporate maximal power training with weight training because the brake catches the weight upon release. It is also very effective because the computer interface gives instant feedback on the power generated by the athlete.

The caveat to this method is that it is still guided resistance, so the proprioceptive and stabilization demands are not very high and it limits exercises to the vertical plane. An even bigger problem is that the system is expensive and currently unavailable in the United States. However, with some ingenuity it is possible to modify a regular Smith machine to be able to catch the bar upon release.

Jump Squat — In this exercise, the athlete rapidly squats down and explodes back up as quickly as possible, aiming to achieve maximal height. With the goal being maximal power production, it is best done with external load.

To determine the appropriate load, it is necessary to first determine the Total System Mass (TSM) as follows: TSM = Body Weight + Max Barbell Weight (Baker pp. 12). For example, if an athlete weighs 200 lbs. and has a maximum squat of 375 lbs., the total of 575 lbs. is the TSM. To determine the optimal training load, calculate 40 percent of TSM (which in this case would be 230 lbs.) then subtract the athlete's body weight (in our example, this results in a training load of 30 lbs.). It is imperative that special care is taken so that loads that are too heavy are not selected. This workout is best performed in rep ranges from 8 to 15 reps for three to five sets. Two times in a seven-day microcycle is sufficient.

Elastic Equivalent — These workouts are designed by pairing exercises consisting of one heavy exercise in the traditional weight training mode followed by an MPT exercise (again, one that allows acceleration over the entire range of the movement). Use no more than three pairs of exercises in a session and only two sessions a week, for a maximum of three weeks. This is very intense work with high nervous-system demands. While this work has the potential to raise explosive power to higher levels, if overused it can dull the nervous system.
Examples would be:

Squat and Jump Squat

Bench Press and Medicine Ball Chest Pass

Hang Power Clean and Stair Jumps with a Weighted Vest

Perform four to six reps of the weight exercises at an intensity of about 75 to 80 percent of max and eight to 12 reps of the elastic equivalent exercise.

Med Ball — To achieve the MPT training effect, it is necessary to use heavier-than-normal medicine balls. If heavy medicine balls are not available, it is possible to use weight plates thrown into a sand or foam pit. Examples of exercises would be triple extension throws backward and triple extension throws forward. (See Figure One) Use three to five sets of six to eight repetitions.

Pendulum Swings — Although this exercise does not technically fit into the MPT mode of training, it can achieve many of the same effects. Hang a heavy medicine ball on a rope suspended from above. The athlete swings the ball away like a pendulum. As the ball returns, the athlete catches it with either one or two hands and immediately accelerates the ball back out. (See Figure Two.)

Kettle Bells (Power Balls) — These are a favorite of the Eastern European throwers. Kettle bells are essentially large, heavy, metal balls with handles. They are not currently available in the United States except in the form of throwing weights for track and field. I often use a power ball instead, which is a plastic ball with a handle for throwing. (See Figure Three) Their advantage is that they can be thrown on any surface without damaging the surface. Power balls vary in weight from 2 pounds to up to 40 pounds.

With these balls, it is possible to execute a clean or a snatch movement and release the ball to achieve maximal power production. It is best to perform these exercises in the range of six to eight repetitions for three to five sets.

Application

To achieve optimum results from Maximal Power Training, it is necessary to have a good overall general fitness base and an extensive weight training background in explosive movements in order to be able to handle the intensity of the work. MPT is probably best utilized during the times in the training year when you want to raise power to new levels. The traditional approach would be to put it at the end of a training program just before the most important competitions occur. That is acceptable, but it may actually be more effective to use it several times through the year, in two- or three-week blocks to raise explosive power. Remember, this method should not be used with beginners. Athletes must have a good strength base and proficiency in their sport before beginning this type of training. ◆

Maximum power training will put the finishing touches on your power development program.

References

Baker, Dan, "Selecting the Appropriate Exercises and Loads for Speed-Strength Development," *Strength and Conditioning Coach,* Vol. 3 No. 2, pp. 8-16, 1995.

Baker, Dan, "Improving Vertical Jump Performance Through General, Special and Specific Strength Training: A Brief Review," *Journal of Strength and Conditioning Research,* Vol. 10, No. 2, pp. 131-136, May 1996.

Wilson, Greg J., Newton, Robert U., Murphy, Aaron J., and Humphries, Brendan J., "The Optimal Training Load for the Development of Dynamic Athletic Performance," *Medicine and Science in Sports and Exercise,* Vol. 23, pp. 1279-1286, 1993.

Wilson, Greg J., "Strength and Power in Sport," *Applied Anatomy and Biomechanics in Sport,* Blackwell Scientific Publications (1994) Carlton, Australia, pp. 110-208.

Leaps and Bounds — Progressing Into Plyometric Training

Plyometric training is not particularly new. The hopping, bounding, and jumping exercises that we now call plyometrics have actually been a part of the training of athletes in a variety of sports for years – it just was not always called plyometrics.

The word plyometrics first appeared in training literature in the late 1960s, when scientific research gave us a fundamental understanding of the elastic properties of muscle and its trainability. This then enabled the practitioner to better understand how to train muscles for explosive power and thus how to more effectively apply plyometrics.

Despite this increase in knowledge, there is still much misunderstanding concerning the application of plyometrics. Because plyometrics has received so much publicity, there have been many exorbitant claims about its effectiveness. At the same time, it has also received much undeserved blame for causing injuries and creating over-training problems.

Plyometric Training is surrounded by many myths and misconceptions. To reap its rewards, one must understand its training demands and appropriate progressions.

What Is Plyometric Training?

Plyometric training is specific work for the advancement of explosive power. Many traditional training programs aim to develop an athlete's maximum strength output, which, when tested in a performance setting, takes 0.5 to 0.7 seconds to exhibit. However, in most athletic events, explosive/ballistic movements that athletes perform do not take that long. Therefore, the premium is on generating the highest possible force in the shortest period of time and reducing or stopping this force at the end of the action. This is the objective of plyometric training and is its primary role in training and rehabilitation programs.

The physiological theory behind plyometric training is to develop efficiency in the stretch/shortening cycle of muscle action. During the stretching (eccentric lengthening phase) of muscle action, a greater amount of elastic energy is stored in the muscle. This elastic energy is then reused in the ensuing shortening (concentric) muscle action to make it stronger. The key is to shorten the coupling time, that is, the time it takes for the muscle to switch from the lengthening/yielding phase to the shortening/overcoming work phase. This leads us to a fundamental principle of plyometric training: the rate, not the magnitude, of the stretch is what determines the utilization of elastic energy and the transfer of chemical energy into mechanical work.

However, it is crucial to understand that plyometrics is only one piece of the training puzzle. The overall goal is to improve the relationship between maximum strength and explosive power. Therefore, plyometrics must be used in conjunction with other power development methods. In other words, plyometrics can only be effective if the athlete also develops basic strength.

Training Loads

When devising a plyometric program, the prime consideration, as with any training method, is determining appropriate training loads. Because plyometric exercises entail a high neuromuscular demand, understanding the training demands of the different activities and allowing enough recovery time is very important in preventing injuries. The following factors must be considered when assigning training demand:

Displacement of Center of Gravity — Horizontal displacement is less stressful than vertical displacement.

Table One: Plyometric Demand Rating Scale

1 = Very Low Stress
Recovery very rapid.
Example: Jump rope or ankle bounce or other low-amplitidue jumps

2 = Low Stress
Recovery rapid. One day required.
Example: Tuck jumps or other similar in-place jumps

3 = Moderate Stress
One to two days for recovery.
Example: Stair jumps or other similar short jumps

4 = High Stress
Recovery slow. Two days required.
Example: Hops or bounds for distance or other similar long jumps

5 = Very High Stress
Three days required. Highest nervous system demand.
Example: Depth jumps or other similar shock type jumps

> **Table Two: Balance & Stabilization Tests**
>
> (These tests are appropriate for use with all ages and should be performed without shoes to test the stabilizers of the foot and ankle)
>
> **1. Static Stand** (Hip Flexed)
>   a) Stand erect on one foot.
>   B) Flex the hip and bend the knee of the non-supporting leg.
>   c) Hold this position for 10 seconds.
>   d) Observe the ability to hold the position with as little shaking or lateral deviation as possible.
>
> **2. Single Leg Squat**
>   a) Squat bending at the ankle, knee, and hip.
>   b) Hold lowest possible position for 10 seconds.
>   c) Observe the depth of the squat and the ability to hold the position with as little shaking or lateral deviation as possible.
>   —Klatt, 1988

This is, of course, dependent on the weight of the athlete and his or her technical proficiency in performing the jumps.

Weight of the Athlete — The heavier the athlete, the greater the training demand. A low-demand, in-place jump for a 150-pound athlete can be a high-demand jump for a 250-pound athlete.

Limb Involvement — Single-support exercises demand more than those involving double support. For example, single-leg repetitive hops are more stressful than repetitive, double-leg jumps.

Speed of Execution — A faster speed of execution for exercises like single-leg hops or alternate-leg bounding will raise the training demand.

External Load — Adding an external load, such as a weight vest, will significantly raise the training demand. It should be noted that external loading will also slow down the movement, thus negating some of the advantages of plyometric training.

Volume — The greater the volume of training, the greater the training demand. Essentially, the volume of training can be high if the intensity of the plyometric activity is low. As a rule, the younger the athlete is-in terms of both training age and stage of physical development, the lower the volume of plyometric activities should be for that athlete.

Intensity — Like volume, greater intensity will raise the training demand. However, it is important to remember that the nature of plyometric exercises inherently demands high-intensity work for optimum return. Generally, the more advanced the athlete is, the greater tolerance he or she has for a larger volume of higher intensity work.

Density — This refers to the number of times plyometrics is repeated within a particular training cycle. The greater the density, the greater the training demand. As a general rule, it is probably inadvisable to include more than three plyometric sessions in a seven-day workout cycle.

Training Age — This is defined as the number of years an athlete has been involved in a formal program. At younger training ages, the overall training demand should be kept low. The exercises or games should be of low nervous-system demand and low motor-complexity. However, it is still possible to get a large number of contacts (volume of activity) with minimum stress through game activities such as jump rope and jumping relays.

> **Table Three: Stabilization Jump Tests**
>
> **1. Hop for Distance:**
>   Appropriate for use with all ages.
>   a) Hop maximum distance. Hold the landing (like a gymnastics landing) for 10 seconds.
>   b) Compare the distance achieved with the right and left legs.
>   c) Check the ability to hold the landing position for 10 seconds.
>   d) Check if the athlete lands bending at the ankle, knee, and hip, incorporating all three joints.
>
> **2. Hop Down (off 12-inch box):**
>   Use only with more mature athletes.
>   a) Hop off the box for maximum distance. Hold the landing (like a gymnastics landing) for 10 seconds.
>   b) Compare the distance achieved with the right and left legs.
>   c) Check the ability to hold the landing position for ten seconds.
>   d) Check if the athlete lands bending at the ankle, knee, and hip, using all three joints.
>
> **3. Repetitive Jump Test:**
>   Maximum effort jumps: appropriate for use with all ages.
>   a) Jump up and down repetitively with a maximum effort jump as rapidly as possible for 30 seconds.
>   b) Observe how rapidly the athlete can switch from eccentric (down) to concentric (up). An excessively long switching time indicates a poor level of eccentric strength.
>   c) Observe how much the athlete deviates from the original starting position. Deviation forward, back, or laterally indicates poor balance and stabilization.
>   d) Count the number of jumps.
>   —Klatt, 1988

To further quantify the task of determining appropriate training loads, I have developed a rating scale. (See Table One) The rating scale is intended as a tool to help monitor the stress of plyometric training, especially as it relates to other activities with high neuromuscular demand, such as weight training and sprinting. The underlying premise is that an activity of high nervous-system demand will take twice the recovery time as compared to a similar load of metabolic work.

Basic Strength

As mentioned above, an athlete must have some basic strength in order for plyometrics to be safe and effective. Some professionals have suggested that prerequisite strength levels, such as the ability to squat two times one's body weight or leg press two and one-half times body weight, are necessary. However, based on my practical experience, research, and the growing understanding of the physiological basis of plyometric training, I feel that these criteria are quite high and, in many cases, unreasonable. When training young athletes, such high strength levels are not necessary or realistic — especially considering the relatively low body weight involved. This is not to say that basic strength is unimportant, rather that it is only one of many factors that must be considered before beginning plyometric training.

A better way to determine if an athlete is strong enough to handle plyometrics is to test his or her stabilization and eccentric strength. To begin to incorporate plyometrics into a training program, the prime concern in order to prevent injury is strength in the stabilizing muscles. Stabilization strength levels can be determined by several simple tests that may be easily administered and interpreted. (See Table Two) If the athlete is unable to satisfactorily perform these tests, then he or she should begin a remedial program of balance and stabilization exercises to bring these qualities up to acceptable standards before plyometrics are incorporated into the training program.

The next concern after stabilization strength is eccentric strength. Especially in more complex, high-volume, and high-intensity plyometric training, lack of eccentric strength can be a limiting factor. Without adequate levels of eccentric strength, rapid switching from eccentric to concentric work becomes very inefficient. It is possible to evaluate eccentric strength through stabilization jump tests and observation of basic jumping exercises. (See Table Three) If on observation, you see an excessively long amortization phase and slow switching from eccentric to concentric work, then eccentric strength levels are not adequate, and the training should be remedial and low in volume and intensity. The specific goal before any emphasis is placed on plyometric training should be to raise the athlete's eccentric strength to an acceptable level.

Skill

Proper execution of the exercises must be continually stressed, regardless of the athlete's proficiency level. In the beginning, it is especially important to establish a sound technical base upon which to build the higher intensity work. Jumping is a constant interchange between force production and force reduction, which leads to a summation of forces utilizing all three joints of the lower body: the hip, knee, and ankle. The timing and coordination of all limb segments will yield a positive ground-reaction force, which results in a high rate of force production. Table Four is a guide for analyzing this skill. The guide is especially valuable when observing the athlete frame by frame on high speed video.

A key element in the execution of proper technique is the landing. The shock of the landing should not be absorbed exclusively by the foot, but rather by a combination of the ankle, knee, and hip joints working together that will absorb the initial shock of landing and transfer that force throughout the body's muscles. Therefore, using all three joints properly is key in allowing the body to use the elasticity of the muscles to absorb the force of landing, which is then utilized in the subsequent movement.

This is not to minimize the importance of the foot strike. The foot strike must be on the full foot in order for the foot to help absorb the shock. It is incorrect to land either completely on the heel or completely on the ball of the foot; such landings will transfer high impact forces through the foot bones and the ankle and knee joints rather than allowing the muscle to absorb the shock. In addition, loud slapping noises created by the landing indicates that the landing technique is incorrect, and the exercise should stop. During repetitive jump tests, the athlete should react to the ground as if it is hot in order to emphasize quickness off the ground.

Upright carriage of the torso is also necessary to ensure proper projection of the center of mass and to avoid undue strain on the lower back. Correct postural alignment is directly related to core (torso) strength. If the athlete is having problems holding the torso erect during the movements, this problem should be addressed immediately through a core-strengthening program.

Table Four: Jumping Skill Checkpoints

1. **Posture:** Check head position and torso position.
2. **Foot Strike:** Must be on the full foot as opposed to the ball or heel of foot; should not land on flat foot.
3. **Landing:** Should e quiet, not loud/slaping.
4. **Leg Action:** Check amplitude and synchronization.
5. **Arm Action:** Must be coordinated.

This program should consist of exercises to strengthen the abdomen and the spinal erector muscles, as well as the rotational muscles of the trunk. The arms make a significant contribution to correct exercise execution in terms of both balance and force production. Research has shown that the arms can enhance the jump by up to 10 percent. It is important for the athlete to learn to use the arms to transfer momentum to the whole body through a correct blocking action. It has been my experience that the torso position and the synchronization of the arms to the exercise are the two aspects of technique that are most difficult for a beginner to master.

Progression

A well-defined progression will go a long way in eliminating some of the inherent risks of plyometric training. The key is not to rush, making sure the athlete masters each step before proceeding.

At the beginning stages, double-leg takeoffs are preferable to single-leg takeoffs and appropriate activities include jumping rope, hop-scotch, sack races, and various jumping and hopping relays to reinforce the natural movement patterns. Within each step, there can be built-in, increasing levels of difficulty, depending on the training level of the athlete and his or her aptitude for learning As the level of mastery of the exercises increases, the amplitude of the movements should also increase. Throughout all stages, it is of paramount importance to place continual emphasis on coordination, fluid movement patterns, and correct motor patterns-regardless of the step in the program.

The following sequential program is one that I have used for years:

1) Landing Exercises: To teach proper foot strike, coordination of the ankle, knee, and hip to absorb shock, and correct body alignment. Have the athlete begin with a simple standing long jump, with a two-foot landing. This should be a sub-maximal jump with an emphasis on "sticking" the landing. The athlete should learn to land quietly on the full foot and absorb shock by bending at the ankle, knee, and hip. Repeat the exercise several times until the athlete is comfortable. Next, have the athlete hop on one foot, with the same objective as above. Repeat until comfortable.

2) Stabilization Jumps: To reinforce the correct landing technique and raise levels of eccentric and stabilization strength. This exercise is very similar to the exercises in Landing Exercises. The main difference now is that the athlete will hold the landing position for a five count before initiating another jump or hop. Repeat until the athlete can stick and hold three jumps, then three hops on each leg for a five count.

3) Jumping Up (Figure One): To teach the takeoff action and the use of the arms. Start with a stable

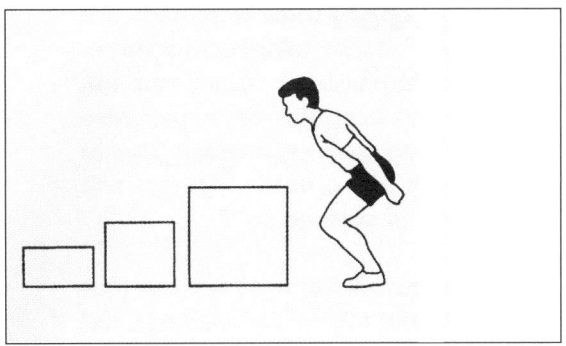

While performing jumping up exercises, the athlete should use a forceful swing of the arms.

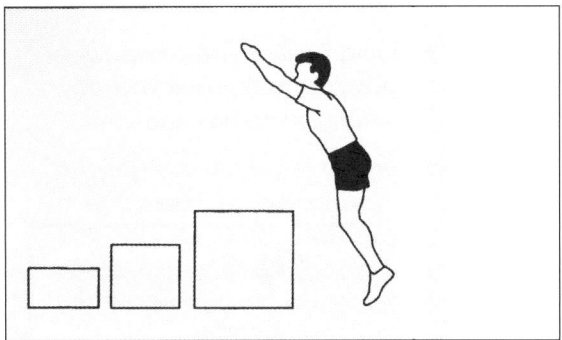

Maintain upright carriage of the torso...

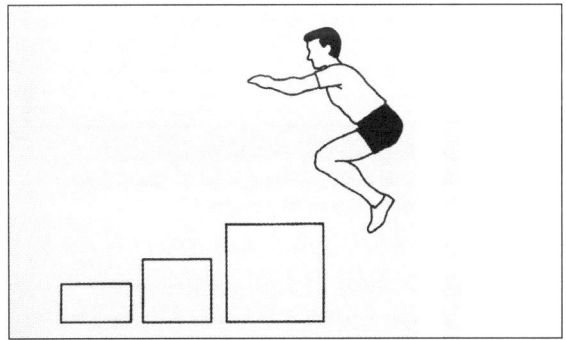

Coordinate the movements of the arms and legs...

bench or box at knee height. Have the athlete jump up onto the bench. Emphasize a forceful swing of the arms to transfer momentum to the whole body. Gradually increase the height of the bench or box to mid-thigh height.

These first three steps should be accomplished within the first teaching or training session.

4) In-Place Bouncing Movements: To teach quick reaction off the ground and vertical displacement of the center of gravity. Begin this step, which should be the start of the second session, by reviewing the first three steps. This will serve as a good warm-up as well as a review of the concepts. This step, step four, entails teaching an ankle-bounce movement, which is essentially like jumping rope without the rope. Then teach a tuck jump, emphasizing quick reaction off the ground while bringing the knees to the chest. With both exercises, the athlete must keep the torso erect. Also check to see if the athlete has the balance and body control to stay in one place—if he or she cannot, then you should not move on. In this session, also teach a scissors jump in order to lead up to the cycling action of the legs that will come into play in the next step. All of the above should be accomplished within the second session.

5) Short Response: To teach horizontal displacement of the center of gravity. Begin by reviewing the previous four jumps. Then start the athlete with three consecutive, repetitive standing long jumps (two-foot takeoff and landing), and progress to five repetitive standing long jumps. Have the athlete do the same exercise going up stairs, jumping onto every other stair. Next, teach the single-leg hop and have the athlete work up to 10 consecutive hops on each leg. Emphasize the cyclic action of both the hopping and the free leg; the action should resemble a single-leg run. Repeat this step for two to three workouts before progressing to the next step.

6) Long Response: to add more horizontal velocity. In this step, teach alternate leg bounding and various combinations of hops and bounds carried out for 10 to 20 contacts. This is as far as most athletes should progress in the first year of training. It is possible to increase the volume, intensity, and complexity of the workouts by adding exercises and combinations of these first six steps.

7) Shock Response: To raise explosive power to the highest levels; high nervous system demand. This is an advanced form of training that requires a large training base. This consists of jumps off of boxes or rebound jumps over hurdles placed at mid-thigh height or higher. The training stress is high. Therefore, this method should be used judiciously, and it is inappropriate for beginners.

Conclusion

Plyometric training has tremendous potential as a training method for all sports that require explosive power. Improperly introduced and taught, it is a high-risk, low-return training activity. To optimize the returns, it is necessary to follow the general guidelines set out in this article.

Reference: Klatt, Lois, PhD., Director of Physical Performance Laboratory, Concordia College. Personal conversation on balance and stabilization testing. ◆

Up, Up and Away — Vertical Jump Improvement

Co-author: Jimmy Radcliffe, University of Oregon

As simple as it sounds, the best means of improving jumping ability is to jump. Advances in technology foster the misconception that specialized equipment and elaborate facilities are required. However, according to current research and our own work with athletes, the opposite has proven true. Strength training without the continual use of specific jumping paradigms yields contrary results. In addition, the actual skills necessary for vertical jumping are difficult to simulate with any type of loaded training method.

Therefore, when training to improve jump height, it makes sense to continually incorporate specific jump training progressions into the strengthening program. This will maintain and improve neuromuscular control. The key is consistent application of simple training methods that address the individual players' strengths and weaknesses.

Elevating your players' vertical jump involves designing a comprehensive program and getting back to basics.

Preliminary Considerations

In designing a program to improve jumping ability, the first step involves considering the following factors:

1) **The demands of the activity.** To improve jumping performance, power must be developed in a rested, non-fatigued state. Therefore, conditioning should be separated from the improvement of jumping power to ensure optimum returns.
2) **The specifics of the activity.** Different sports and even different player positions have different requirements with regard to jumping. The number, intensity, and types of jumps can differ greatly. For example, a soccer midfielder may average 10 maximum-height jumps per game, while a forward in basketball will perform a high number of sub-maximum and maximum jumps from many different angles. For any sport, the number of maximum jumps and sub-maximum jumps the player takes during a game should be determined and then used as a baseline in developing the program.
3) **The qualities of the individual athlete.** Age is the first factor to consider. Younger athletes should be given a less intense program than older, more mature players. There are also gender considerations: female athletes often need more emphasis on strength training than male athletes. A third area to take into account is basic leg strength levels of the athlete. An often-overlooked area where strength deficiencies limit jumping ability is the core, which consists of the hips, abdomen, and lower back. Finally, bear in mind the type of jumper you are working with: a quick jumper requires only a slight bend at the ankle, knee, and hip to achieve maximum height and generally will thrive on work that requires less overload and features more explosiveness. A slower strength jumper must get more bend in the hips and knees in order to jump higher and will thrive on more strength work and a larger workload.
4) **The pattern of injuries.** Postural defects can predispose the athlete to injury if additional training stress is added. Common jumping injuries are lower back strains, patellar tendonitis, Achilles tendonitis, shin splints, and plantar fasciitis. Any of these injuries can significantly limit improvement in the vertical jump.

Jumping Mechanics

In order to realize optimum results from a jump improvement program, it is important to understand correct jumping mechanics. Perhaps the best visualization is to imagine the body as having three large springs at the hip, knee, and ankle .(See Figure One) To give these springs energy, they must be compressed. This is accomplished by crouching down, which stretches the muscles that cross these three joints. This downward movement activates the stretch shortening cycle (SSC) of muscle action (also called the plyometric effect). The net result

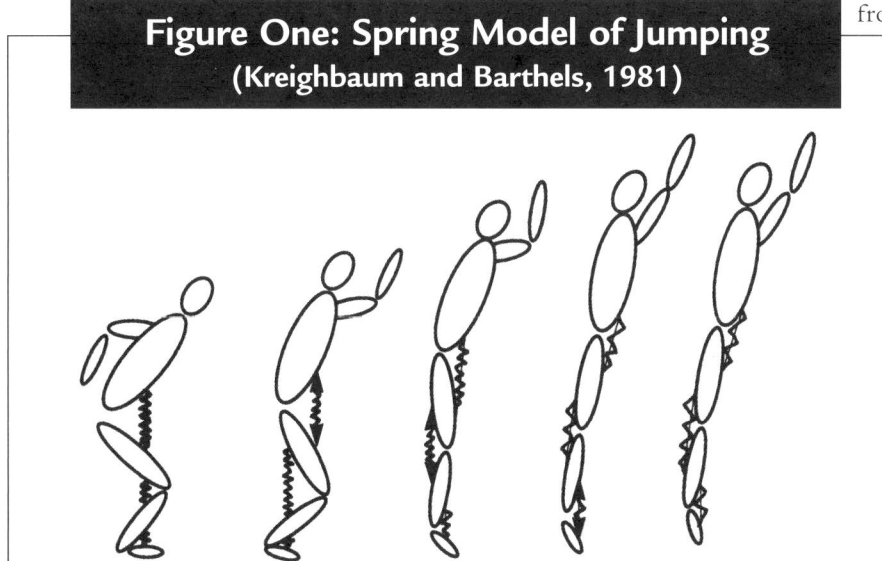

Figure One: Spring Model of Jumping (Kreighbaum and Barthels, 1981)

Table One: Program Overview

	High School	College
Off-Season Training To Train	Strength Training: 1 x BW, 3-4 x ER Plyometrics: 3x Core Work: 4x	Strength Training: 1 x BW, 4 x ER Plyometrics: 3x Core Work: 4x
Pre-Season Training To Compete	Strength Training: 1 x BW, 3 x ER Plyometrics: 2x Core Work: 4x	Strength Training: 1 x BW, 3 x ER Plyometrics: 3x Core Work: 4x
In-Season Competition	Strength Training: 1 x BW, 3-4 x ER Plyometrics: 1x Core Work: 2-3x	Strength Training: 2 x ER Plyometrics: 1x Core Work: 3x

BW= Body weight exercises; ER= External resistance exercises; 1x, 2x, etc. = Number of training sessions per week

is a stronger contraction of the muscles that cross the hip, knee, and ankle. The objective is to put force into the ground in order to raise the center of gravity as high as possible. Once this compression occurs, the springs begin to uncoil in a sequential pattern as follows:

1) **Arm Swing:** The action of the arms serves to raise the center of gravity as high as possible before take-off and to transfer momentum to the rest of the body to increase ground reaction force.
2) **Trunk/Hip Extension:** The muscles that cross the hip are the largest and strongest muscles of the body. Therefore, they have a tremendous potential to contribute to the height of the jump. That is why the training program emphasizes hip extension exercises and medicine ball work.
3) **Knee Extension:** This area has traditionally received the most attention in jump improvement programs. It is important, but not nearly as important as hip extension.
4) **Ankle Extension:** The last segment to come into play. Strengthening the ankle is actually more important in injury prevention than it is in force production.

Another way to look at the takeoff to a jump is as a chain reaction, where one segment begins to decelerate as the next segment begins to accelerate. The essential aspect of this sequence is the efficiency of movement centered around the timing and coordination of the muscles of the different segments of the body. In the second half of the jump, the landing is the opposite of the takeoff, with the ankle, knee, and hip bending sequentially to absorb force.

Testing Jumping Ability

Jumping tests are intended to provide a performance profile of the athlete's jumping ability in order to direct the training program. The tests should simulate the jumping requirements of the sport and also be included in the training program so that incremental progress can be easily assessed.

1) **Vertical Jump:** Determine standing reach with dominant hand, then jump as high as possible (starting from a standing position), recording the highest height of the hand. The score is the difference between the reach and the height touched. Take the best of three jumps.
2) **Step-Close Jump:** Step out onto one foot, bring the back foot in line with the front foot, crouch, and jump. Take the best of three jumps. The result should be four to six inches higher than the vertical jump.
3) **Running Jump:** This is best performed on a basketball court. Start running at the free throw line, take off on one foot and touch as high on the backboard as possible. Take three jumps off each foot (to compare the best jump off each foot). The result should be higher than the previous vertical and step-close jumps.
4) **Repetitive Hops:** Hop five times on the right foot and five times on the left foot, striving for both height and distance, and recording the total distance. Compare the results to identify any strength difference between the two legs.

Taken together, these tests give a profile of the player's overall jumping ability and thus will allow you to develop a specific direction for the training program. If deficiencies are detected in any one area, then that area must be emphasized until it is up to the standard of the other tests. The best time to correct deficiencies is in the off-season and early in the athlete's career. It is particularly important to address the balance between the two legs as indicated by the single-leg hop test. If there is more than an 18-inch difference between the legs in the repetitive hop test, then the deficient leg must be worked on to bring it closer to the strong leg. This is important for injury prevention as well as performance enhancement.

Program Design

As in designing any type of exercise program, there must always be a balance between volume, intensity, and frequency. To improve an explosive quality like jumping, intensity is the most important component, while frequency and volume will depend on the athlete, the time of the training year, and the player's level of development.

Table Two: High School Plyometric Program

Off-Season

MB Toss for Height:	(4Kg Ball) 3 x 10
MB Overback Throw:	(4Kg Ball) 3 x 10
Jump Rope:	10 x 50
Jump and Stick:	5 x 5
Hop and Stick:	5 x 5 each leg
Tuck Jump:	3 x 10
Lateral Jumps:	3 x 10
Jump Up:	3 x 10
Squat Jumps:	5 x 10
Vertical Jump:	3 x 10 (Measure each jump)
Step Close Jumps:	3 x 10
Rubber Band Jumps:	5 x 10
Drop Jump:	3 x 5

Pre-Season

MB Toss for Height:	(4Kg Ball) 2 x 10
MB Overback Throw:	(4Kg Ball) 2 x 10
Jump Rope:	10 x 50
Jump and Stick:	5 x 5
Hop and Stick:	5 x 5 each leg
Tuck Jump:	3 x 10
Jump Up:	3 x 10
Squat Jumps:	4 x 10
Vertical Jump:	2 x 10 (Measure each jump)
Step Close Jumps:	2 x 10
Rubber Band Jumps:	3 x 10
Drop Jump:	3 x 5

In-Season

MB Toss for Height:	(3Kg Ball) 1 x 10
MB Overback Throw:	(3Kg Ball) 1 x 10
Jump Rope:	8 x 50
Jump and Stick:	5 x 5
Hop and Stick:	5 x 5 each leg
Tuck Jump:	3 x 10
Lateral Jump:	2 x 10
Squat Jumps:	2 x 10
Vertical Jump:	1 x 10 (Measure each jump)
Step Close Jumps:	1 x 10
Rubber Band Jumps:	2 x 10

Jumping ability should be developed throughout the entire training year. Frequency and volume should be highest during the off-season and pre-season, but quality work must still be completed during the competitive season. In monitoring athletes' jumping abilities at the University of Oregon, we have found that a year-round program (that continues into in-season training) is the best way to see measured improvement during the competitive season. Another important consideration in program design is the amount of aerobic work that is included in the program. Experience has shown that large amounts of aerobic work are detrimental to vertical jump improvement. The best results occur when the emphasis is placed almost entirely on explosive activities with only the minimum of aerobic work necessary for warm-up or cool-down.

Three more tips to keep in mind:
1) The training program must be practical, meaning that it can be accomplished within the context of the time and facilities available.
2) It must be personal and individualized as much as possible in a team setting to that athlete's level of development and performance profile.
3) It must be motivational, so that the athlete can relate to it and see progress and results.

Training Methods

A total jump improvement program must include strength training, extensive core work, and plyometrics. The following is an outline for the areas of strength training and core work and details the actual plyometric program. As a guideline, strength training should consist of body weight exercises and weight training. Body weight exercises may include: the single leg squat, body weight squat, lunge, step-up, and jump squat. Weight training exercises (i.e., with external resistance) may include: the squat, single leg press, lunge, walking lunge, step-up, high step-up, hang clean, pull down, pullover, combo curl & press, and incline bench press. Core work may include: an abdominal circuit, medicine ball throws, and medicine ball rotations and twists.

Plyometric training is specific work to improve jumping power by training the stretch shortening cycle of muscle action. This work must be sequenced with the other conditioning components as well as sport specific practice because it is a significant training load that can have a high risk of injury if not used properly. Progress from single response repetitions to multiple responses with a pause and then to multiple response work without pauses. The following are descriptions of the plyometric exercises outlined in Tables Two and Three:

Medicine Ball Toss for Height — Hold ball at chest. Dip quickly down to a semi-squat position, immediately extend arms and legs, and release the ball so that it travels straight overhead as high as possible. Allow ball to bounce on the ground, catch it, and repeat as rapidly as possible.

Medicine Ball Over the Back Throw — Start with ball overhead, swing the ball down between the legs while flexing the trunk and the knees. Immediately reverse direction and throw the ball over the back as far as possible while extending the legs, trunk, and arms.

Jump and Stick It — Hold landing position five counts.
Hop and Stick It — Hold landing position five counts.
Jump Rope — Set of 50 jumps in various combinations.
Tuck Jump — Jump in place, pull the knees to the chest.
Lateral Jumps — Double leg back and forth over a line.

Ice Skater — Side to side pushing off one leg onto the other and repeat.

Rubber Band Jump — Use a 48-inch rubber band for resistance.

Jump Up — Jump up onto a box or a table that is mid-thigh to waist high. On take-off there must be rapid extension of the hips and knees and a quick explosive pushing off from the ground with simultaneous blocking of the arms into a flexed landing position on the box. Use the following starting positions:

- **Static Squat** — Start in a semi-squat position with the feet positioned hip-width apart and the arms back (in a position ready to thrust forward and up).
- **Counter Move** — Start with an upright stance with the same foot positioning as the previous position. Perform a quick flexion into a semi-squat position followed by an immediate take-off.
- **With a Step** — One foot remains in the previous position under the hip, while the other foot is placed behind. The knees are bent and the weight is shifted to the forward foot to avoid any "rockerstep" action. The back foot creates momentum upon push off for the subsequent take-off.
- **Lateral Step & Bound** — Positioned approximately one and one-half steps directly to the side of the normal take off position, push off with the outside foot and lead with the inside leg into a lateral move to a two-foot take-off from the original take-off spot.
- **Squat Jumps** — Repetitively squat down and jump as high as possible.
- **Standing Vertical Jump** — Nonrepetitive, maximum-effort jumps measured.
- **Step-Close Jumps** — Maximum-effort jumps measured.
- **Step Back & Jump** — To practice jumping from an unfamiliar position.
- **Shuffle/Slide Jumps** — Jump and touch as high as possible on the right side of the backboard. Land and shuffle to the middle of the key, jump up and touch the rim. Land and shuffle to the left, jump, and touch as high as possible on the left side of the backboard. Repeat back to the right for a total of six jumps. That is one set.
- **Drop Jump** — Step off a 12- to 18-inch-high bench onto both feet and jump as high as possible.

Putting the Pieces Together

The program overview (See Table One) is intended to give a broad picture of how all the training methods fit together relative to the individual player's level of development. The high school program is geared toward athletes ages 15-18 with the objective of reinforcing correct jumping mechanics and introducing some complex exercises. The college program is for athletes ages 18 and up with the objective of maintaining the volume, but raising the intensity of training and individualizing the program.

Tables Two and Three are specific plyometric programs for each level, broken up into the time of the training year. These two regimens are formatted as middle-of-the-road programs and can be altered depending on the specific athlete or team. Take into account the factors outlined in each section of this article to make the program work for your athletes. ◆

References:

Bobbert, Maarten F, and van Soest, Arthur J., "Effects of Muscle Strengthening on Vertical Jump Height: A Simulation Study," *Medicine and Science in Sports and Exercise,* Vol. 26 #8, 1994, pp. 1012-1020.

Kreighbaum, Ellen and Barthels, Katherine M., *Biomechanics — A Qualitative Approach for Studying Human Movement.* Burgess Publishing Company, Minneapolis, Minnesota, 1981, p. 408.

Table Three: College Plyometric Program

Off-Season
Exercise	Sets/Reps
MB Toss for Height:	(4Kg Ball) 4 x 10
MB Overback Throw:	(4Kg Ball) 4 x 10
Jump Rope:	5 x 50
Jump and Stick:	5 x 5
Hop and Stick:	5 x 5 each leg
Tuck Jump:	3 x 10
Jump Up:	4 x 10
Squat Jumps:	5 x 15
Step Close Jumps:	3 x 10
Rubber Band Jumps:	5 x 10
Drop Jump:	3 x 10

Pre-Season
Exercise	Sets/Reps
MB Toss for Height:	(4Kg Ball) 3 x 10
MB Overback Throw:	(4Kg Ball) 3 x 10
Jump Rope:	10 x 50
Jump and Stick:	5 x 5
Hop and Stick:	5 x 5 each leg
Tuck Jump:	3 x 10
Jump Up:	3 x 10
Squat Jumps:	4 x 12
Step Back & Jump:	3 x 10
Side Step & Jump:	3 x 10
Rubber Band Jumps:	3 x 10
Drop Jump:	3 x 10

In-Season
Exercise	Sets/Reps
MB Toss for Height:	(3Kg Ball) 2 x 10
MB Overback Throw:	(3Kg Ball) 2 x 10
Jump Rope:	8 x 50
Hop and Stick:	5 x 5 each leg
Tuck Jump:	2 x 10
Squat Jumps:	2 x 10
Vertical Jump:	1 x 10 (Measure each jump)
Step Close Jumps:	1 x 10
Rubber Band Jumps:	2 x 10

Getting Gait Right

Running is not only a fundamental motor skill, but also a crucial ingredient of nearly every sport that takes place on land. Whether running is a direct sport component or a vital training activity for a given student-athlete, improving running mechanics can significantly improve his or her sport performance.

Running skill, like any motor task, is teachable and trainable. Using a systematic approach, you can help even someone who seems to be hopelessly gangly improve his or her gait.

There are two goals in improving running mechanics: First, to learn to optimize ground reaction forces — the point of contact where all the forces are concentrated for a relatively brief period of time. The second goal is to achieve optimal efficiency, which means that less energy is expended to complete the same task. Not only will improved running mechanics translate to an ability to do more work, but it will also result in greater speed and a reduction in injuries.

Know the Laws

In running, as in all movement, there are three constants: the body, gravity, and the ground. While the specifics of each may change, all three are always there, and the athlete is always at the mercy of their basic laws. For example, the athlete must work within the laws of biomechanics and physiology. The body works in predictable patterns with all systems blending together to produce a desired movement pattern. We can manipulate the body and make corrections to its movement patterns, but only within its natural confines.

Gravity is the force we must overcome to propel the body forward. As gravity pushes the body down into the ground, the body must resist this force and then overcome it to propel itself up and forward. The ability to reduce the effects of gravity through shock absorption is a very important component of sound running mechanics.

Finally, improving running mechanics is directly dependent on the ability to use ground reaction forces effectively. This is the force that reacts to the push transmitted from the foot to the ground and propels the body. At speeds as slow as three to six meters per second, which is essentially a range from a slow jog to a run, the ground reaction forces are two to three times bodyweight.

Contrary to the marketing hype for various commercial programs, equipment is not necessary to improve running mechanics. Improving running mechanics is really about optimizing the relationship between the body, gravity, and the ground. Treadmills and other exotic apparatus will only interfere with the body's ability to move naturally.

A Systematic Approach

As with any fundamental skill, a systematic approach to improving running mechanics will yield optimum results. The system I have developed is the PAL System, for posture, arm action, and leg action. These are the three main areas of emphasis in running. This system provides a context to analyze movement as well as a step-by-step teaching progression. It can also be used to design a criterion-based progressive approach to getting someone back to a normal gait pattern following an injury.

Improving running mechanics is the single best thing athletes can do to improve their game in almost every sport played on land.

Posture is the most important of the three components — it has been my experience that if posture is improved, arm action and leg action will follow naturally. Posture should reflect the alignment of the body from the point of foot contact with the ground to the top of the head. The reference points for this alignment are the head, trunk, hips, knees, ankles, and feet.

The image and cue for good posture is that of "running tall." After the start and acceleration, the sensation should be of running only at the very point of contact with the ground: lighter, taller, and with less ground contact time than during the acceleration phase. Good posture strongly reinforces this feeling.

Arm action serves two primary functions: the arms assist with balance as well as provide a strong propulsive force during the acceleration phase. The arms also play a vital role in helping to control the rhythm of running. The direction of the swing of the arms should result in linear motion. Running, like all other movements, involves movement in all three planes — transverse, frontal, and sagittal with sagittal being the dominant plane of motion. But while some rotary, as well as side-to-side, movement of the arms is necessary to counteract rotation of the body and the mass of the legs, this movement should be minimal. Proper running mechanics requires controlling — not eliminating — rotational movement and side-to-side sway.

The amplitude of the arm action will vary with the speed of the run. The shorter and faster the run, the greater the amplitude of the arm action. Arm action will also be exaggerated at other times, such as when propelling the body up a hill.

The optimum leg action is to have the foot contact the ground as close under the body's center of gravity as possible. This will yield the most efficient stride. The amplitude of the leg action as reflected in the knee lift and stride length will vary with the speed of the run. Good running mechanics requires an optimum interplay between stride length and stride rate (frequency). Each person has an optimum stride length in relation to his or her leg length and the distance he or she is running.

Making the Big Fixes

When observing the runner in an effort to improve running mechanics, observing from several vantage points will provide better analysis. Watching from only one vantage point will not allow the observer to see all aspects of the stride. Running should be viewed from the side, front, and rear. From the front and rear, have the athlete run along the edge of a line while you watch where his or her feet strike in relation to the line. He or she should run along the line—hitting the line with the insides of the feet—not on the line or crossing over the line.

Have the athlete run with different gait patterns—long strides and short strides, no arm action and exaggerated arm action, and with different foot strikes—forefoot, flat foot, and heel first. Observe how he or she accommodates or compensates. This is important to help you get the feeling of what is right for that specific individual. At first, don't coach the athlete or make corrections, just observe the movement.

To correct running mechanics, it is best to use the Fault / Reason / Correction paradigm. First, identify the fault in the mechanics. Then find the reason for the flaw and correct it. Table One is a checklist of common running mechanic skill faults to look for and correct. This is by no means an exhaustive list.

Look at the big things first in the context of the PAL System. Get a sense of the flow of the action before looking at specific considerations. Focus on smaller pieces of the puzzle only after global considerations have been addressed. This is in concert with the whole / part / whole concept of motor learning — start with the whole action (in this case, running), then look at the parts. Decide what parts need attention. Design task-oriented drills or movements that will reinforce the correction of those parts. Rather than focusing on the fault you are trying to correct, give the athlete a task to achieve that will correct the fault. Allow him or her to explore and solve the movement equation. Then, as soon as possible, relate the drill back to the whole action.

In designing drills to improve running mechanics, consider the following questions:
- Why drill? Drill to reinforce correct patterns or to change or improve incorrect patterns.
- What drills? The drills should be as directed and specific as possible. A few drills clearly defined and well chosen are better than a large number of general drills that dance around the issue. Beware of drilling for drills' sake — make sure the drills are truly reinforcing correct mechanics that relate to an individual's specific needs. A common pitfall to avoid is designing drills that break the movement into too many component parts. Always relate the drill back to the whole action of running.
- When should drills be done? The optimum time for learning is when the athlete is fresh and fully recovered from any previous training stress. Therefore, drills are best done near the start of a training session.
- How to do the drills? Based on the objective of the respective drill, make sure the athlete correctly executes it.

Drills alone may not be enough to significantly improve running mechanics. Improved strength can also be a big factor. Segmental weakness can contribute to poor mechanics, especially in the core. Therefore, it is important to couple any program that attempts to improve running mechanics with a sound strength training program that utilizes multi-joint and multi-plane exercises.

Target the Training

Running mechanics vary with and must be adapted to the speed of the run. A sprint has different demands than a distance run. The most visible change along the continuum from a sprint to a long distance run is in the amplitude of the movement. A sprint demands longer stride length, greater air (flight time), and shorter ground contact time, as well as vigorous arm action, higher knee lift, and a forefoot foot strike. Efficiency is not as much of a consideration as is the pure production of power.

A distance run will have shorter strides, much shorter flight time, longer ground contact time, a mid-foot to rear-foot strike, and lower, more economical arm action. The longer the distance run, the more important efficiency becomes.

Improving running mechanics is not a quick fix. Like any other motor skill, it is teachable and learnable, but it demands constant attention and fine-tuning. It requires body awareness, balance, and good basic core and leg strength. Each running step is a step toward ingraining a new motor pattern or reinforcing an established pattern.

By working to improve running mechanics, athletes will improve their balance, speed, and endurance, and help to prevent injuries. Improving running mechanics yields a greater range of benefits than improving practically any other single skill. ◆

After the start and acceleration, the sensation should be of running lighter, taller, with shorter ground contact time.

Resources

The following resources are useful for those seeking further information on running mechanics:

Gambetta, V., Winckler, G. *Sport Specific Speed—The 3S System*, Gambetta Sports Training Systems: Sarasota, Fla. 2001.

Gambetta, V., Odgers, S. *Straight Ahead Speed* [video], Gambetta Sports Training Systems: Sarasota, Fla. 1995.

Running Mechanics Checklist

The following is a checklist of running mechanic skill faults that need to be screened when observing an athlete. This is by no means an exhaustive list, but it provides a good idea of what to look for.

Posture
Leaning backward
Bending forward at the waist
Excessive side-to-side sway
Head position — back or forward

Arm Action
Arms swing across the midline of the body
Arm carriage:
    Too high
    Too low
Abbreviated arm action
Excessive arm action

Leg Action
Foot strike—exaggerated forefoot or heel contact
Stiff hips
No knee lift

In a Blur — Basic Speed Development

How to Develop Sport-Specific Speed

In games like football, basketball, soccer, baseball, and tennis, success or failure often comes down to a "moment of truth," a point in the contest when the offensive player outmaneuvers the defense, or the defense shuts down an offensive drive. And in most instances, these moments are determined by the players' speed and their ability to apply that speed to crucial game situations.

Traditional thinking dictates that "sprinters are born, not made." While this is true to the extent that it is not possible to be a world-class sprinter or record-breaking running back without genetic endowment, sport science and coaching practice have done much to refute this limiting statement.

Speed is both a biomotor quality and a motor skill. As a biomotor quality, it is defined as the ability to perform a specific movement in the shortest possible time. In a motor learning context, it is a learnable skill that can be enhanced through sound, motor-learning principles. Ultimately, it is only through the practice of such motor skills and intense training that any genetic endowment can reach its highest potential level.

Overall, sport-specific speed encompasses the ability to start quickly from all different positions, accelerate to top speed in the shortest time possible, change direction, and stop rapidly under control. The goal in this chapter is to provide a conceptual framework of speed as it applies to sport performance; the principles discussed here are applicable to all sports where speed is a key aspect of performance. The crucial element is the ability to apply that speed to the specific demands of the sport or position.

Speed Components

Speed training includes many interwoven components, each of which must be understood by the coach before a training program is implemented. These components include: the energy and nervous systems, body composition, power, range of motion, and leg speed.

Much discussion occurs on the role of the energy systems in speed development, but this component is actually quite clear-cut. The primary energy demand for speed comes from high-energy phosphate stores, which are alactate anaerobic. The lactate anaerobic system has very little, if any, effect on speed performance and the aerobic system is not a factor at all in terms of actual speed. It is much more important to emphasize the nervous system, which is heavily taxed by the high-intensity demands of speed. Within the nervous system, also called the "central command" system of the body the motor units, are the smallest functional units of neuromuscular system. Sprinting is essentially the recruitment and innervations of the appropriate motor units and the proper synchronization of firing patterns between motor units. This results in alternating responses of ultra fast excitation and relaxation.

It is also significant that there is a close correlation between the percentage of fast-twitch fibers and speed of movement. Although fiber type is genetic, training can have a tremendous effect on the recruitment and utilization of the correct fibers. Too much slow endurance work will recruit the intermediate fibers to assume the properties of slow-twitch fibers, which will adversely affect peak power production. Conversely, high-intensity work can train the intermediate fibers to take on the properties of fast-twitch fibers.

Speed can be significantly improved through a systematic program.

Overall, the nervous system must receive careful consideration when designing a training program, as it is the dominant influence on speed performance. Care must be taken to design exercises and training sessions that facilitate the recruitment of the appropriate motor units to produce the greatest rate of force production in the shortest possible time. Due to improper training design and frequent competition, many athletes work in a constant state of nervous system fatigue. A general training rule is to allow twice the recovery time for nervous system work as for energy system work. Failure to observe this guideline results in poor performance and frequent injuries to muscles and tendons.

Anthropometric characteristics such as height, weight, and leg length are not significant factors in speed development. Research has found that optimal stride length at absolute speed is usually 2.3 to 2.5 times the athlete's leg length, no matter if the legs are short or long. Body composition, however, does play a significant factor in speed — the leaner the athlete, the more efficient the performance. Therefore, excess body weight carried as fat is detrimental to performance.

Speed improvement is definitely linked to improvement in power, which is the capacity to produce the greatest amount of force in the shortest possible time. The fastest athletes spend less time on the ground and have longer strides, which they are able to repeat with greater frequency — all of which are directly related to strength and power. Maximal contractile strength is required at the start and during the early stages of acceleration, up to a speed of 7.5 meters/second. At that point the requirement begins to shift to elastic strength, which is dependent on the stretch-shortening cycle of muscular action.

The ability to move the appropriate joints through a

large range of motion at high speeds is also essential. This is often confused with static flexibility, a factor that has little relationship to performance. Speed work demands a large amplitude of movement at the shoulders, hips, and knees, and that requires dynamic flexibility. The efficient application of these large ranges of movement is related to joint stabilization and balanced strength development.

Leg speed, the final component of speed, is a careful blend of the two components of the stride-length and frequency, both of which can be improved through properly directed training. The most essential aspect of the stride with respect to game situations is the ability to control it, which is more closely related to the frequency. A relatively long stride that is adapted well to the straight-ahead running demanded by the 100-meter dash is not always adaptable for games where the demand is on quick starts and equally quick stops and where reaching top speed is seldom achieved. (It is important to point out that 100-meter speed is not a liability, but simply must be adapted to the specific speed requirements of the game.) A slightly more compact stride emphasizing leg speed allows for more control and change of direction, as well as quick starting and stopping.

A Training Program

Improving speed should begin quite early in a player's career. In fact, in order to develop speed to its ultimate potential, speed training should begin by the ages of eight to twelve — the so-called "skill hungry years." At this stage, frequency of stride is especially important to develop with effective training methods being those that stimulate frequency of movement and increase speed with a focus on quality and intensity. This should occur in a playful environment with an emphasis on games that demand short, intense, all-out bursts of speed. It is also important to note that this training should be done in an alactate environment of games, specific movement exercises, and short relays. The role of maturation cannot be underestimated in the perfection of the motor skills of speed. Many technical problems in the acquisition of speed that occur in young athletes are due to a lack of physical maturity; i.e., poor joint stabilization strength and trunk (core) strength, which usually manifests itself as poor posture. As the athlete matures, gains strength, and improves body awareness, many technical faults will be self-corrected.

At the high school and college levels, sprint mechanics should first be reviewed, and preferably mastered, and then followed by sport-specific running workouts. To accomplish this, it is necessary to use a mixture of drills and exercises. Some exercises should coincide exactly with how the movement is performed, while other exercises may emphasize only part of the total movement. These latter drills usually consist of drills that break the sprint stride into its component parts and seek to apply that as a movement.

In order to teach proper sprint mechanics, there are three elements to consider—posture, arm action, and leg action — which should be analyzed and corrected in that order. I have found that this is an easy concept for the athlete to grasp in order to correct mechanics.

Posture is the alignment of the body, which is dependent on the situation. In acceleration, there is more of a pronounced lean to overcome inertia. In top speed, there is a more erect posture. In either case, you should be able to draw a straight line from the ankle of the supporting leg through the knee and the hip, then another straight line through the torso and head. In acceleration, the angle between these two lines will be between 40 and 45 degrees, and in absolute speed it will be around 85 degrees.

Arm Action refers to the amplitude, or range of motion, of the arms, which is essential to acceleration

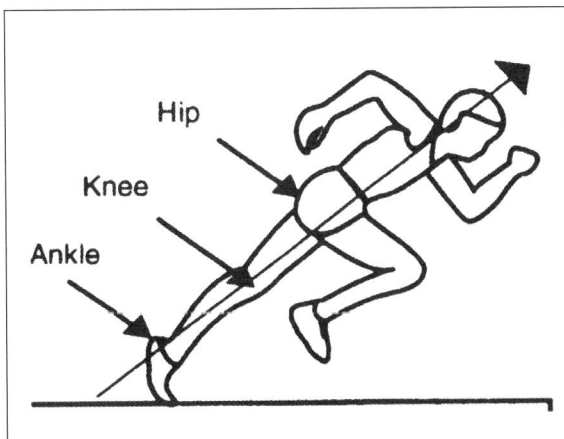

Figure One: During early acceleration, the emphasis is on backside mechanics, which focuses on extending the ankle, knee, and hip in a triple extension.

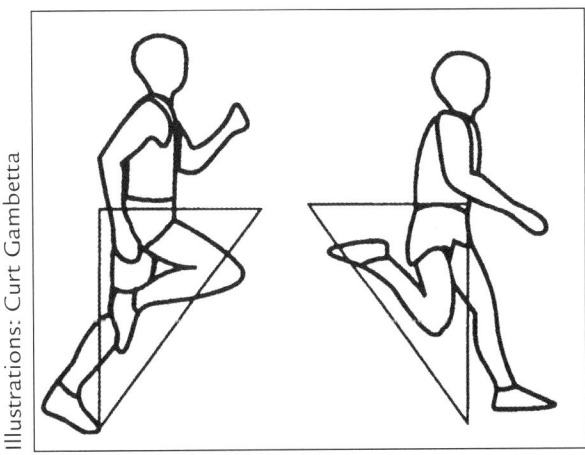

Figure Two: At maximum speed, there should be a balance between frontside and backside mechanics.

and control of the stride. In acceleration, there is a more piston-like arm action, which will smooth out as top speed is achieved.

Leg Action is the action and orientation of the hips and legs relative to the torso and the ground. For quick starts, it involves extending the ankle, knee, and hip to produce the greatest force possible against the ground. For quick stops, it entails bending the ankle, knee, and hip to reduce force and to control the stop.

Each area of spring mechanics has a profound effect upon the other two. If one is off, then you will notice a compensation in the other two. It has been my experience that they generally occur in the enumerated order: Poor posture will lead to compensations in arm action and then a reduced amplitude of movement with the legs.

After the athlete has learned proper sprint mechanics, divide speed into the following phases to provide a context for evaluation as well as a logical division for training process. Workouts should imitate the planting, cutting, stopping, and starting from different positions that are required to play the athletes' sport:

Start — The goal of the start is to overcome inertia and get the body into an efficient position to accelerate as soon as possible. The start includes the reaction to the primary stimulus, whether it is the ball, the player, a sound, etc., and the subsequent drive from the starting position. There is some confusion between reaction and reflex. Reaction time is the time necessary for the muscles to respond to the starting stimulus. A reflex, however, is an involuntary action that occurs below a conscious level and is not under the athlete's control. An example is touching a hot object and immediately pulling back the hand. Reaction, on the other hand, is a conscious, voluntary action that the athlete can control. It is trainable and can be improved through skill work and conditioning that involves recognition of the correct stimulus and execution of the correct pattern of movement.

An efficient start is dictated by starting stance, which is determined primarily by the strength level of the individual athlete as well as body dimensions, the sport, and the position. Tremendous contractile strength is necessary both to generate the high forces necessary to overcome inertia and to push against the ground in the first four to six strides.

Acceleration — This is the rate of change of velocity that allows the athlete to reach maximum velocity in a minimum amount of time. The goal in acceleration is to advance toward top speed as quickly and efficiently as possible. Because of the posture of the body, which is in a pushing/driving position due to the degree of lean necessary to overcome inertia and get the body moving, the emphasis in early acceleration is on backside mechanics. This is defined as the action of the legs that occurs behind the center of gravity as a result of extending the ankle, knee, and hip. It is this extension which results in the pushing action against the ground over the first six to eight strides until a more upright posture is achieved.

During this phase, the head is in line with the torso and the torso is in line with the legs. There should be no bending at the waist in an attempt to increase body lean; all lean should occur from the ankles.

Maximum Speed — This phase, in which the athlete is running at the highest velocity, is a minor factor in sport performance for most game situations. Also termed "fast coordination," this phase demands the highest levels of neuromuscular coordination.

Speed Endurance — This is defined as the ability to hold the highest percentage of maximum speed for the duration of the event, and is highly related to good sprint mechanics as well as alactate anaerobic capacity.

Lateral Speed and Agility — This refers to kinesthetic awareness, spatial awareness, change of direction, and deceleration/stopping.

A Workout Plan

In constructing a workout plan for speed development, use a chart or table format that incorporates training distance, training volume, intensity, and frequency. (Please see Table One for examples of speed development training methods.) An overview of a 16-week program is as follows:

Weeks One and Two: Mastering the basics.
Weeks Three and Four: Refining technique and correcting individual weaknesses.
Weeks Five to Eight: Adding new drills and raising the volume of work.
Weeks Nine to Twelve: Emphasizing resistance-running drills.
Weeks Thirteen to Sixteen: Raising the intensity and dropping the volume to bring speed qualities to a peak.

Speed workouts can be integrated into all aspects of a normal practice in the following manner:

- As part of the warm-up, with an emphasis each day that rotates between starting and acceleration, lateral speed and agility, and absolute or top-end speed.
- During the actual skill part of practice, with one aspect of speed as a specific objective.
- During post-practice time with an emphasis on short speed endurance and good mechanics.

There are an amazing number of drills to improve speed, and many successful sprint schools have made extensive use of them. While many of these drills can be beneficial, I feel that it is still important for the coach to understand the purpose and application of each drill, as many are designed for specific strength, not sprint mechanics.

Table One: Speed Development Training Methods

Normal Conditions
Objective: To train all qualities of speed without resistance or assistance.

Methods:
Starting Work:
5 x 5 Yard Start — Right Foot Forward
5 x 5 Yard Start — Left Foot Forward
5 x 10 Yard Start — Jump and Go (off each foot)
5 x 10 Yard Start — Yard Scramble Out

Acceleration Work:
40 x 40 meter with a Standing Start — 3 min recovery
6 x 60 meter Hill Sprint — 3 min recovery
6 x 20 meter Block Starts

Speed/Quickness Work:
10 x 10 Yard Burst — 1 min recovery
5 x Quarter Eagle Right
5 x Quarter Eagle Left
5 x Scramble Up
5 x Scramble Up with Reaction To Ball
5 x 40 meter Accelerations — 2 - 3 min recovery

Absolute Speed Work:
6 x 30 meter with 20m Flying Start - 4 min recovery
4 x 50 meter with Ultra Speed Pacer - 4 min recovery
4 x 60 meter Variation Run (sprint 20m/Float 20m/sprint 20m)

Speed Endurance Work:
2 sets of 5 x 50 meter at 95% with 1 min recovery — 5 min between sets
1 x 120 meter at 90% - 5 min recovery
1 x 150 meter at 95%

Lateral Speed & Agility Work:
Resisted Conditions
Objective: To develop specific strength in order to improve stride length and/or acceleration. The training effect can be altered depending on the weight of the external load or the degree of incline of the hill.
  Methods: Weight Vest, Ankle Weights, Uphill Sprints, Sled or Tire Pull, Parachute, Sand, Stairs.

Assisted Conditions
Objective: To develop specific strength in order to improve stride frequency. The training effect can be altered depending on the degree of incline of the hill or the method of towing.
  Methods: Downhill Sprints, Tubing, Towing, Ultra Speed Pacer, Tailwind.

Keep in mind that sprinting is a natural, rhythmic, flowing activity that should not be made mechanical. The best way to improve speed is to sprint, and the farther away the training activity is from the actual sprinting, the less the application it will have to improving speed. Therefore, it is important not to deviate too far from the whole action. Drills should be a means to an end, not an end in themselves.

Lastly, remember that work and correction of mechanical faults should always be done in a non-fatigued state. Too often, the athlete is asked to make changes when the nervous system has already been maximally taxed or, even worse, when the athlete is bathing in a pool of lactate from too much lactate anaerobic work.

Sprinting is the most natural of all physical skills, yet it is still a highly complex motor skill that can be improved significantly through proper training. Hopefully, some of these concepts will help you to develop a sport-specific speed development model that is appropriate for the athletes with whom you are working. ◆

References

Bruggemann, Gert-Peter, and Glad, Bill. "Scientific Research Project at the Games of the XXIVth Olympiad — Seoul, 1988, Final Report," *New Studies in Athletics*, Supplement, 1990.

Dick, Frank. *Sprints and Relays,* British Amateur Athletic Board, 1987.

Radford, Peter. "The Nature and Nurture of a Sprinter," *New Scientist*, August 2, 1984.

Winckler, Gary. "Principles of Application for Enhanced Sprint and Hurdle Performance," 1990.

Getting Up To Speed — Acceleration

When evaluating athletes, we often test their speed to determine their performance potential. However, in most sports, it is not speed but acceleration that determines effectiveness. US soccer star Mia Hamm, for example, may have never won a 100-meter dash, but her ability to accelerate to the ball is one of the attributes that makes her so outstanding.

Seldom in team sports do athletes go beyond the acceleration phase. However, they are constantly changing speeds — accelerating to a new offensive or defensive position on the field or court.

Acceleration is part of the conceptual framework of the whole speed-development process. The good news is that this component of speed is highly trainable. In fact, it may be the most trainable component of speed.

To understand the various concepts of acceleration, keep in mind the ultimate finished product: the world-class sprinter. The principles and mechanics of the highly trained sprinter are the same for all sports that require overground propulsion. At the same time, however, it is necessary to design training that is specific to the needs of the athlete relative to the sport.

The Concepts

What exactly is acceleration? Acceleration is the rate of change of velocity. Optimally, it allows the sprinter to reach maximum velocity in a minimum amount of time. Most sprinters, whatever their level of performance, reach maximum speed between 30 and 60 meters from the start in a 100-meter race. In the Seoul Olympics for example, the male 100-meter finalists reached maximum speed between 50 and 60 meters. (Bruggemann, 1990)

There are many components to developing acceleration that all work together. Here's how they break down:

Mechanics of Acceleration — Acceleration mechanics should be evaluated and trained in the context of posture, arm action, and leg action (PAL):

Posture describes the alignment of the body, especially the head and trunk. Posture is dynamic and changes with each step from the starting position through top speed. It is important that "lean" comes from the ankle, not the waist.

Improving acceleration can do wonders for your athletes' performance. It is a skill that can be significantly improved.

Arm Action addresses the position and amplitude of movement of the arms and hands. The arms help to produce force and aid in balance so that force is properly applied against the ground. The emphasis during acceleration is on driving the arms down and back to help apply force against the ground.

Leg Action focuses on the foot, ankle, knee, and hip. Leg action relative to acceleration is a driving phase characterized by the feeling of pushing back behind the body during the initial steps. (Dick 1987) The emphasis here is on backside mechanics — what occurs behind the body. The pushing action occurs from the start through the first four to six steps, after which the athlete assumes a "hips tall" position. See Figure One for a look at a proper pushing triple extension position.

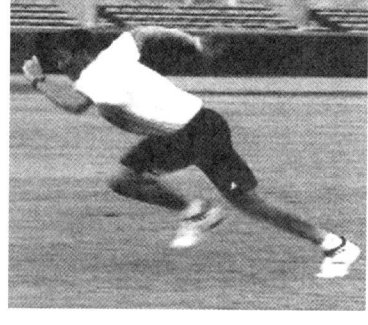
Figure One: Triple Extension

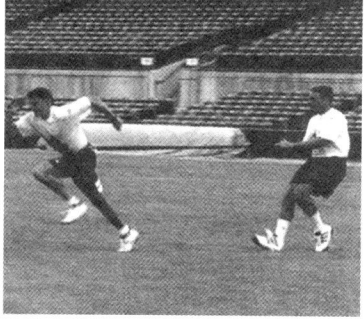
Figure Two: Harness Sprints

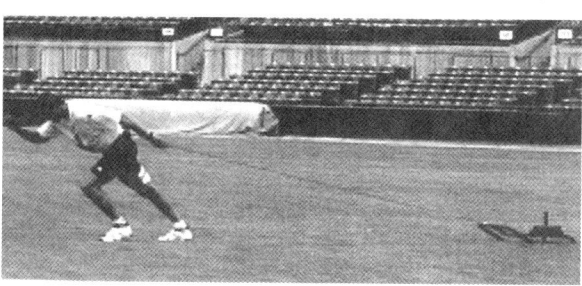
Figure Three: Sled Pull

Each aspect of acceleration mechanics (posture, arm action, leg action) has a profound effect upon the other two areas. If one is off, there will be a compensation in the other two. It has been my experience that problems generally occur in the enumerated order: poor posture will lead to compensations in arm action and a reduced amplitude of movement in the legs.

Pattern of Acceleration — To ensure correct force application and proper transition to top speed, it is necessary to have a proper pattern of acceleration. The pattern consists of each succeeding step increasing in length until full stride length is achieved.

Most young athletes try to take steps that are too long, thinking that they will get to top speed sooner. In effect, the opposite occurs: they end up stumbling and reaching, which slows them down and puts them at greater risk of injury. Steve

Myrland, former Strength and Conditioning Coach at the University of Wisconsin, uses the analogy of someone driving a stick-shift trying to go straight from first gear to fifth gear. Inevitably, the car will stall. The same thing happens to the athlete who tries to go too fast too soon without shifting gears.

After the start of a sprint, the athlete accelerates by increasing both stride length and stride frequency. Ultimately, sprint performance is determined by an optimum combination of these factors. Of the two, stride frequency is more limiting in sprint performance. It is influenced by the pattern established in the first few steps.

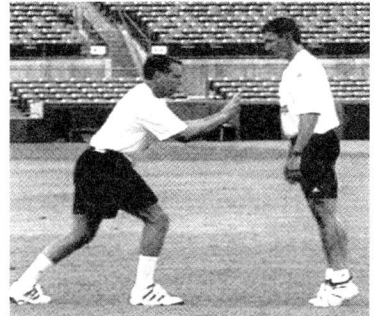

Figure Four: Drop and Go

The sprint stride consists of two parts: the flight phase and the ground contact phase. During the initial drive from the blocks, horizontal forces predominate. Ground contact times, as studied by Anti Mero in Finland, decrease over the first strides. As the race progresses, vertical velocity plays a bigger role, which is manifested by the sprinter being airborne 50 to 60 percent of the stride cycle. This flight time can be thought of as the time it takes for the legs to cycle properly in anticipation of ground contact.

Force Application — The goal, as well as a key coaching point in all of this, is to create a positive shin angle, which allows for proper force application and control of the stride throughout the distance being run. This is an angle of the shin to the ground where the foot contacts the ground behind the center of gravity on the first two steps and then as close as possible under the center of gravity after that.

The opposite is a negative shin angle, where the foot contacts the ground in front of the center of gravity. This results in a braking action, which causes athletes to pull themselves over the ground-contact foot. The body is highly inefficient in this action, as well as more prone to injury.

To create a positive shin angle on the first step (and each succeeding step), it is imperative to get the foot down as quickly as possible — you can only apply force while on the ground. The key is to impart as much force to the ground in the shortest possible time. In the early phase of acceleration, when ground time is longer and flight time is shorter, visualize the airborne foot stepping over the foot/ankle. As the "hips tall" position is achieved and flight time increases, the cue is to step over the calf. Once top speed is achieved, flight time is at its greatest, and the cue is to step over the knee.

Training

Acceleration improvement is closely linked to improvement in power. Greater strength results in the ability to produce higher amounts of force more quickly, which decreases ground contact time, enhancing both stride frequency and length. The strongest sprinters spend less time on the ground and have longer strides which they are able to repeat with greater frequency.

Maximal contractile strength is required at the start and the early stages of acceleration up to 7.5 m/sec. It is best trained with resistance work including weight training, harness running, sled pulls, and so forth. After that point, the requirement begins to shift to elastic strength, which is dependent on the stretch-shortening cycle of muscular contraction. The elastic phase is trained with plyometric work like hurdle jumps, hopping, and bounding, where ground contact is minimized.

When designing a training program, keep in mind that the high-intensity demands of sprinting primarily tax the central nervous system (CNS). Therefore, care must be taken to design exercises and training sessions that facilitate the recruitment of the appropriate motor units to produce the greatest rate of force production in the shortest possible time. Due to improper training design and/or frequent racing, many athletes are in a constant state of nervous system fatigue. A general training rule is to allow twice the recovery time for CNS work as for energy-system work. Failure to observe this results in poor performance and frequent injuries to muscles and tendons.

Acceleration training should begin early. It is appropriate to begin at the ages of 8 to 12, during the so-called "skill hungry years," with tag games and playful drills that promote good acceleration mechanics. At this crucial stage, emphasize training methods that stimulate frequency of movement and increase speed with a focus on quality and intensity. Use a variety of starting positions to stimulate proprioceptive development. Such training should be short, intense, and playful.

The role of maturation, however, cannot be underestimated in the perfection of any of the motor skills involved in acceleration. Many technical problems that occur in young athletes are due to weak joint-stabilization strength and core strength resulting from a lack of physical maturity. As the athlete matures, gains strength, and improves body awareness, many technical faults are self-corrected through growth and development.

In designing a training week to include acceleration training, I have found it best to include two days of acceleration, usually on Monday/Thursday or Tuesday/Friday coupled with plyometric and strength training. This pattern will ensure enough time for recovery. Skill work and correction of mechanical faults should always be done in a non-fatigued state. Too often the athlete is asked to make changes when the nervous system has already been maximally taxed and there is little chance of correct movement being learned.

Drills

The best way to learn how to accelerate is to accelerate. Therefore, it is important to not deviate too far from the whole action.

To accomplish this, it is necessary to use a mixture of first and second derivative exercises. First derivative exercises coincide exactly with how the movement is performed in the total movement. A harness run with light resistance would be an example. Second derivative exercises coincide only with part of the total movement. One example is the stick drill.

It is important that the coach understand the purpose and application of the drill. Many drills are designed for specific strength but do nothing to teach or reinforce correct acceleration mechanics. Sprinting is a natural, rhythmic, flowing activity that cannot be made mechanical. A few drills done correctly are much better than a whole menu of drills done for their own sake.

Stick Drill — This drill teaches the proper pattern of acceleration. Essentially, the drill consists of accelerating from a standing start and hitting a series of sticks placed on the ground at predetermined distances with each step. The spacing of the sticks determines the pattern of acceleration.

The drill was introduced to me by Pat Reid, a Canadian high jump coach, who had seen the East German women sprinters use it in their training. Their races were always characterized by high stride frequency and an excellent pattern of acceleration. Unfortunately, we did not know any of the details of the placement of the sticks so we arbitrarily placed them at 12-inch increments. This resulted in increased turnover and a somewhat improved pattern of acceleration, but it did not allow good force production. University of Illinois track coach Gary Winkler then worked out the spacing of the sticks based on stride length out of the starting blocks and leg length of the athletes so that the distance between sticks progressively increases with each step, thus forcing a correct pattern and application of force against the ground.

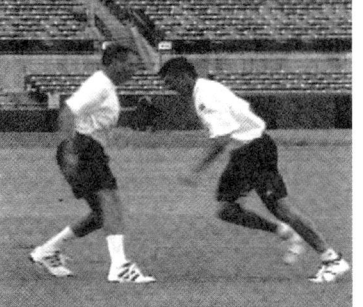

You will need to experiment with the spacing based on the leg length and developmental level of your athlete. A good starting point is to place the second stick 15 centimeters from the first and increase the distance between each consecutive stick by 15 centimeters, so that the spacing would be 15 cm, 30 cm, 45 cm, 60 cm, etc. For the non-track athlete, use only five or six sticks; for the sprinter it is advisable to use 10 sticks. Be sure that the athlete is applying force back against the sticks, not running over them in a pitter patter fashion. Use this drill as a teaching aid, and be careful not to overuse it.

Harness Sprints — Use the harness to facilitate good posture rather than overload. Use only moderate resistance, just enough so that the athlete can feel the extension and pushing action. Too much resistance will slow the action and alter the mechanics of acceleration. (See Figure Two)

A good variation is to release the harness after five or seven steps to create a contrast effect. This also serves to test the athlete's posture and overall mechanics. If the transition is smooth out of the release, then everything is mechanically sound.

Sled Pull — Use the sled to overload. (See Figure Three) Observe the "10-percent rule:" the resistance of the sled should not slow the runner down more than 10 percent of the best time of the distance being run.

Drop and Go — This is a good drill to put the body in the proper posture for acceleration and to create a positive shin angle. (See Figure Four) The athlete starts in a hips tall position, falls forward, and is caught by the partner. The lean position is held for a count of one and the partner drops the runner. The runner immediately sprints out.

Scramble Out — The athlete starts in a prone position. On command, the athlete sprints out as fast as possible. This drill will put the athlete in a pushing position as well as force the athlete to use the arms. (See Figure Five) Whether your athletes are speeding to a goal line, away from a defender, or toward an opponent, improving acceleration will enhance their performance. Overall, take the time to implement appropriate drills for your athletes, and don't overtax the central nervous system. ◆

References

Bruggemann, Gert-Peter, and Glad, Bill, "Scientific Research Project at the Games of the XXIVth Olympiad - Seoul 1988, Final Report," *New Studies in Athletics*, Supplement, 1990.

Dick, Frank, *Sprints and Relays*, British Amateur Athletic Board, 1987.

Winkler, Gary, "Principles of Application for Enhanced Sprint and Hurdle Performance," (unpublished manuscript), 1990.

Multi-Directional Speed

When we think about training for speed, we conventionally think about players running straight ahead at full speed. But when we think about the movement of players in a game, many other images come to mind — a shortstop moving quickly to her right, a wide receiver running under a ball, a soccer goal keeper making a diving stop.

If we take a moment to analyze them, we see that the vast majority of sports movements are not in a forward line, but actually involve quick starts and stops. In fact, beyond the skill of the sport an athletes' success is dependent on the ability to start and stop quickly and fluidly. This is also known as lateral speed and agility, or LSA.

Just as we can teach a player to become a better hitter, teaching a player to improve LSA is very possible. All it takes is an understanding of some basic concepts about the subject and implementing the drills that are most effective for the different players' positions.

What is LSA?

Lateral speed and agility is the ability to react to the proper stimulus, start quickly and move in the correct direction, change direction if necessary, and stop quickly to make the play. The goals of LSA training are to: 1) improve quickness 2) improve body control (keeping the hips over the feet) and 3) prevent injury through proper movement mechanics.

The program is based on the concept that fundamental movement skill must precede sport specific skill. These fundamental movement skills are the basis for more complex movements. Complex, sport-specific movements are composed of a series of linked fundamental movement skills. If the players have a rich repertoire of motor skills to draw from, it is easier to acquire sports specific skills, and they are less prone to injury because they are prepared for all situations. Along with fundamental movement skills, LSA involves incorporating the following components into your drills:

Reaction — This is the stimulus that triggers the movement. The stimulus can be visual, auditory or kinesthetic. Reaction should be worked on daily because it does not induce any fatigue — it just requires concentration.

Starting — Starting to move involves a triple extension of the ankle/knee/hip in order to produce force and get the body in motion. This is a key component of almost all LSA drills.

First Step — The goal is to create a positive shin angle in order to produce force and get the body moving in the correct direction with the least effort possible.

Drop Step — This is used when it is necessary to

Wheel Drill Protocol

One-Step Drill
1. Start with a correct stance with the hands and arms in the appropriate position.
2. Step out low and fast, holding that position for a three count. Return to the starting position. Stay low when returning to the starting position.
3. Repeat two times at each spoke of the wheel.

Three- and Five-Step Drill
1. Start with a correct stance with the hands and arms in the appropriate position.
2. Start by driving out low and fast for three steps, then progress to five steps. Break down into a fielding position and hold for a three count.
3. Walk back to the starting position and repeat.
4. Add a ball, then add different reactions to the ball (do not progress to step four until the previous steps are mastered).

Baseball Example, Position-Specific Emphasis
Catchers: Start in a catching stance. Simulate throwing off the mask on spokes 4, 5, and 6 as in pop fly situations. Use spokes 1, 2, 3, 7, and 8 for blocking ball simulations.
Middle Infield: Emphasize spokes 3, 7, 1, 2, and 8 in that order.
First Base: Emphasize spokes 1, 3, 7, and 6 in that order.
Third Base: Emphasize spokes 1, 7, 3, and 4 in that order.
Outfield: Emphasize spokes 4, 5, 6, and 1 in that order.
Pitchers: Emphasize spokes 1, 3, and 7 in that order.
Baserunners: Emphasize spokes 2, 3, and 7, in that order.

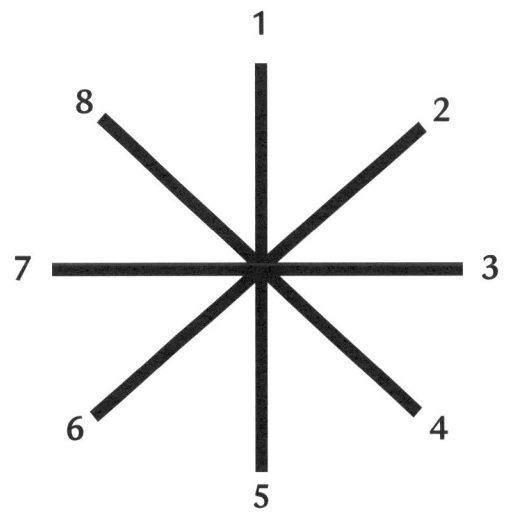

move backwards, either diagonally or straight back. The lead foot moves back diagonally or straight back. The push-off is from the back foot.

Footwork — This is the ability to move efficiently, lightly, and quickly. Control of gravity and positioning the center of gravity are the major objectives of proper footwork.

Change of Direction — Just as the name implies, this is the ability to rapidly stop and reverse direction.

Body Awareness/Balance — Control of the center of gravity is key, which essentially means orienting the hips to the base of support.

Stopping — Stopping is bending the ankle/knee/hip in order to effectively reduce force.

The Wheel Principle

All lateral speed and agility training is based on the Wheel Principle, which is the basis of 3S System Sport Specific Speed®. The best way to visualize the Wheel Principle is to think of the player as the hub of the wheel with eight spokes extending off this hub. These eight spokes define the eight different possible directions of movement she or he may go in. The idea is to train the player in those directions she or he will be moving the most during competition. For example, an outfielder or defensive back should be working mostly on the directions of spokes 4, 5, 6, and 1, while catchers and soccer players need to be able to move in all directions of the wheel. The purpose of the wheel drill is to:

- teach correct mechanics of the stance and first step;
- develop functional strength in the legs at the correct angles as required by the respective positions; and
- teach correct stopping mechanics.

Correct mechanics of the stance and the first step are the most overlooked element of LSA, but they are critical to improving first step quickness and the ability to move laterally. Also keep in mind that control of the center of gravity begins with a proper stance or starting position.

The following are descriptions of the key components of correct stance:

Foot Position/Weight Distribution — Toes should be pointed straight ahead with the feet parallel and the weight evenly distributed over the full foot. Somehow, the misconception has arisen that it is necessary to be up on the toes. This is inefficient in that the foot must come back down to the ground to initiate movement. This is a wasted motion, which costs valuable time. The weight should be distributed in a pattern of approximately 75 percent to the forefoot and 25 percent to the rear foot in order to allow multi-directional movement.

Base of Support — The base should be about shoulder width apart to facilitate movement in any direction.

Angle of Ankle/Knee/Hip — It is important to have proportional flexion (the amount the body angle is bent) at the ankle, knee, and hip so that on first movement the center of gravity is projected in the proper direction, not up or down. The ability to achieve this position will vary with strength, flexibility, and to a certain extent, body proportions.

Trunk Inclination — A slight forward angle is desirable so that the chest is just over the knees. The angle of the trunk should form a parallel line with the shins.

Head Position — The head should be in line with the torso and stay in that position. Moving the head

---

Sample Drills

Here are some specific activities to help to improve LSA:

Jump Rope: This is perhaps the most basic of all LSA improvement activities. A lost skill among the younger athletes of today, jumping rope works hand/foot and hand/eye coordination. It is best to develop a routine that the player can use daily as a warmup for other footwork drills. A basic routine is: double leg jumps, stride jumps, crossover jumps, single leg jumps, and finish with combinations. You can do these in a series with a prescribed number of jumps for each exercise or for a set time period for each exercise.

ABC™ Ladder: This is a great footwork tool that does much of the teaching for you. It is an apparatus that looks like a ladder placed on the ground. The player is challenged and rewarded by correct technique. The key to using the ladder effectively is to understand that the goal is optimum speed, which is defined as speed that can be controlled. There is a tendency on these drills to go too fast, which results in the athlete being out of control and unable to finish a drill. The emphasis should be on getting the feet back down to the ground quickly.

Ball Drop: The partner stands an appropriate (for the level of ability) distance away. The partner drops the ball from head height. The player executing the drill must react and catch the ball before the second bounce. Make the drill more difficult by lowering the distance of the drop or moving farther away.

Z Ball: This is a small rubber ball with round protrusions that cause the ball to take unpredictable bounces. An athlete can work solo against a wall or with a partner. It is very challenging!

Low Box Quick Step: Use a four-inch high box of sturdy construction approximately 30 inches square. Step on and off the box as quickly as possible. Continue the drill until the rhythm falls off. The drills can be done straight ahead, side to side, or with a combination of boxes.

significantly can have a profound effect on the center of gravity and a negative effect on balance.

Arm and Hand Position — The arms and hands should be positioned to aid in the first movement.

It is also important to understand the mechanics of the First Step. The first step should be of appropriate length in order to create a positive shin angle and properly apply force against the ground. A positive shin angle entails the foot hitting slightly behind the center of gravity — thereby allowing the large powerful hip extensors to work. A negative shin angle is created by a long first step in which the foot is relatively far in front of the center of gravity. This forces the player to try to pull him or herself over the foot and is not an advantageous position for force production.

The direction of the first step must be in the intended direction so that the player can gain, not lose, a step. The most common footwork error is the false step or mis-step. This occurs when the player steps back before stepping forward or otherwise steps away from the intended direction of movement.

The type of first step is determined by the distance of the required movement:

Crossover Power Step — This is appropriate when the distance to be moved is relatively great, such as a base runner sprinting for second. The lead foot remains stationary and the back foot crosses over the lead foot. The push-off is from the original lead foot.

Open Step — This is appropriate when the distance to be moved is short or a quick reaction is required, such as moving toward a ground ball or making a tackle. The lead foot steps out with the push-off from the back foot.

Jab Step — This can also be used when the distance is short and a quick reaction is required. This is a backward movement of the lead foot relative to the center of gravity.

Developing LSA Skills

How should these movement skills be developed? The optimum order of development is to first learn the movement without any regard to speed. Then increase the speed of the movement while paying particular attention to maintaining the precision of the movement. The third step is to change the movements or do them under slightly different conditions. Then, finally, follow with specific sport skills based on the movement skill.

Another important consideration in designing drills is the idea of "game speed." As soon as the drills are taught and mastered, then they have to be practiced at the speed you'd do them in a game situation. Practicing slower, in predictable patterns of motion, will lead to what is referred to as a speed barrier. The nervous system becomes used to the same stimulus, which in this case is slow. Then, when called upon to react and move faster, the nervous system is incapable of doing so because the slow pattern has been ingrained. The best time to do movement drills is at the beginning of practice. Every day, the drills should progress from fundamental movement skills leading to sport specific movements. This allows the drills to be used as a warmup — players are both warming up and practicing skills at the same time! It also means drills will be done while the athlete is fresh, which allows optimum results. The total time devoted to LSA drills should be about 15 to 20 minutes per day. Choose three to five drills daily. Be sure to allow enough rest between drills so that quality is maintained, and always remember to have your athletes learn to execute the action correctly, then add the speed component. ◆

Sprint Drills — the Gerard Mach Way

I am going to try to lend a bit of a historical perspective to the evolution of sprint drills as I have seen them during my coaching career. I must emphasize that this is my perspective and opinion based on discussion and observation, as well as my coaching experience. I was first introduced to the Mach drills in 1975 by a group of Canadian athletes training in Santa Barbara, Calif. They showed me the drills and gave me an article on the drills written by the originator of the drills, Gerard Mach, who was the National Sprint & Hurdle coach of Canada. I was immediately attracted to the drills because I could see logic and a system to their application. (This logic and systematic approach to their application has been lost over the years, even in Canada). Superficially, they did not appear that different from the drills that Bud Winter (Coach at San Jose State University and the coach of Tommy Smith, Lee Evans, et al) had taught for years, but after reading Mach's article, there was a logical sequence that was not there with the Winter drills.

I began to use the drills with good results, but I felt that I needed to find out more about the drills and how they fit into the whole system of sprint development. In 1976, the Canadian National Track & Field Team had a training camp in southern California. At this camp, I was able to see Mach coach for several days. This gave me a better depth of understanding of the drills and their application. I also saw how they were applied in hamstring rehab when I watched Coach Mach work with a 400-meter runner who had pulled his hamstring three days previously. In 1977, I met Dr. Al Biancani, who was the coach at Cal State University, Stanislaus. He had apprenticed under Mach. Al was very generous to share his knowledge of the Mach system and his interpretation with me. This was a tremendous help in understanding correct technique on the drills, coaching cues, as well as their place in the whole system. In January 1978, I was able to attend a presentation by Gerard Mach where he spent three hours detailing the development of the Mach Polish Sprint School from his experimentation as an athlete to the application with athletes like Andzej Badenski and Irena Szewinska. It was an epiphany. It was an incredible system. As I look back, he was far ahead of his time. The system and concepts that he had articulated in the 1950s are those concepts that every good sprint coach uses today.

A cornerstone of his system was the "A", "B", and "C" drill series. The drills were also designed to enable the sprinter to get the repetition of work necessary to prepare to actually sprint in the adverse weather conditions that occurred in the winter in Poland. In presentations, he always pointed out that he did not have the good weather that the American sprint coaches in the west and south enjoyed, so he had to come up with alternatives.

Mach broke the stride into its components' parts: knee lift, foreleg action, and the push-off through the drills. The "A" Drills were designed to work the knee lift component. The "B" Drills were designed to work on foreleg reach or pawing action. According to Mach: all exercises with leg extension and active down are special exercises to strengthen the hamstrings. The marching and skipping exercises were designed to develop the technique required for body lean, arm action, high knee lift, leg extension, and keeping the center of gravity high, but did not emphasize the strong driving forward or push forward action." (Page 6, *Sprinting & Hurdling School* by Gerard Mach, CTFA 1977). The "C" Drills were designed to work on push-off and extension.

Gerard Mach is the originator of the modern system of sprint drills designed to improve specific strength and posture for speed.

My interpretation, from discussions with Gerard Mach and Biancani, as well as my extensive use of these drills over the years, is that their primary benefit is not as technique drills. They are drills that specifically strengthen the muscles in postures and actions that are similar to those that occur during the sprint action. It is through strengthening in the specific positions that technique is improved. I consider them posture drills, specific strength drills, and functional flexibility drills. The technical benefit is ancillary. These drills do have a place in a sprint training program if they are properly taught and constantly coached. Incorrect execution and repetition can ingrain bad habits.

One of the biggest faults of the "A" series of exercises is the emphasis on knee lift at the expense of impulse off the ground. The knee lift occurs as a result of what happens on the ground. On the drills, the knee should not be pulled off the ground, but driven down to create a quick strike on the ground, which will result in knee lift. Another fault that I see in execution of the drills is the rate of execution. Mach emphasized that the drill should be executed at "three steps per meter." He also emphasized the necessity of correct arm action on the drills. Too many times I see athletes doing the drills with very passive arm action, which is incorrect.

Each drill is subdivided into a march action, a skip action, and a run action. This was designated by the subscript as follows:
    A_1 = Marching
    A_2 = Skipping
    A_3 = Running

B_1 = Marching
B_2 = Skipping
B_3 = Running

The progression was from marching to skipping to running. The drills were used daily as part of warm up. They were actually used as workouts to emphasize either power speed or strength endurance. They were also used for rehab after hamstring pulls. For workouts, the drills could be done at less than 10 repetitions, less that 10 meters, and less than 10 seconds. This was termed "Power Speed." Mach would also add resistance to the drills in the form of a sandbag or a weight vest. If this was the case, then the drills were designated as "Power Speed Mixed." If the drills were done longer that 20 meters, more than 10 reps and more than 10 seconds in duration, they were designated as "Strength Endurance." If resistance was added to this, then it was termed as "Strength Endurance Mixed." Irena Szewinska was reported to have executed series of 200 Meter A_2s. I personally have used A_2 and A_3 for 4-6 x 50 meters with a weight vest (10% body weight) with developmental athletes.

The drills are a great lead in to teaching hurdles. The lead leg action is actually a "B" action, the trail leg is a "C" action, closely coupled with an "A" action. Another aspect of the drills that picked up from Mach that I do not see applied very often is to link the drills to acceleration. For example, execute an A_3 for 10 meters and change it over to an acceleration of 30 meters. The goal here is to work a particular component of the stride and to immediately place it into the context of the whole action.

In summary, Gerard Mach was a genius. His work has stood the test of time. If we understand that the drills are part of a complex used to develop the sprinter, hurdler and jumper, then they do have a place in the daily preparation of the athlete. As a side comment, it is interesting to note that Tom Tellez, coach of Carl Lewis and Leroy Burrell, did not believe in the use of drills. The bottom line is that that there are many roads to Rome! ◆

Speed Ways

Improving running speed and quickness is a complicated process that must address the biomechanical, physiological, and neurological components of training. Overall, it entails learning correct sprint mechanics, practicing the components of speed (i.e., the start, acceleration, maximum speed, speed endurance, and lateral speed and agility), and adding new drills in order to keep the athlete motivated.

To accomplish these objectives, it is best to use a variety of methods. Fortunately, there are a number of products now on the market that can be used as tools for improving speed. However, selecting the appropriate equipment for your specific athletes can sometimes be confusing.

Generally, most all the devices for speed improvement fall into two categories: resistance-based methods and assistance-based methods. Adding resistance to a drill increases the force necessary to move at a fast speed, while adding assistance allows the athlete to increase speed of movement. The ultimate goal in a speed training program is an optimum combination of resistance and assistance that works to improve stride components without compromising correct sprint mechanics.

Before reviewing the various products, I will first briefly discuss the objectives of the resisted and assisted methods of training:

The Resisted Method, which slows the athlete's movement, enhances motor learning by controlling the athlete's action. This enables the athlete to develop the kinesthetic feel for the optimum positions for force application. In other words, it allows the athlete to get comfortable with the position of the foot behind the center of gravity. Similarly, resistance will also improve sprint mechanics by allowing the athlete to feel the proper placement of the feet, which is necessary to achieve a mechanically efficient technique. This is especially important at the start and in acceleration. Lastly, this method of training will develop specific strength in the muscles used during sprinting, which is especially important in starting and acceleration work and can also aid in injury prevention and rehabilitation.

The Assisted Method allows the athlete to develop the kinesthetic feel of running at a faster velocity than the athlete is normally capable. This forces the athlete to adapt his or her mechanics to a higher level of speed, tuning up the temporal or timing mechanism by developing the necessary "fast coordination" to fire the muscles at the high rate of speed. This method will also teach the athlete to run in a more relaxed manner.

Speed improvement devices generally fall into two categories: those that use resistance and those that provide assistance.

Instead of trying to have the athlete run at a speed that is faster than normal, the athlete can run at 90 or 95 percent of top speed and allow the assisted method to provide the other five to 10 percent — which will result in greater relaxation at top speed.

One final note on these training methods—always observe the 10 Percent Rule in order for the method to be as movement- and velocity-specific as possible. No more than 10 percent of the athlete's body weight should be used when providing overload for resistance, and the time should not be slowed down by resistance or increased by resistance by more than 10 percent.

The devices mentioned below can all be used to train for speed and quickness. My critique of each one is based on my personal opinions reached in using the devise and my evaluation of the research that is currently available.

The speed chute consists of a parachute attached to a belt that is placed around the athlete's waist. It uses the resistance method of training and is most effective at improving posture while sprinting. Some brands are adjustable in size in order to vary the resistance; some simply can be purchased in different sizes. This device is not completely realistic for use in starting and short acceleration work, however, because there is a lag time between when the athlete starts to accelerate and when the chute completely fills with air. Because of this lag time, maximum resistance is achieved later, which sets up an unrealistic pattern of resistance. One way to lessen this problem is to have a partner hold the chute open before sprinting so that it fills sooner.

An important feature to look for in the chute is a belt that can be easily released so that the athlete can use the contrast method. This entails running at a set distance with the chute on and then releasing it to feel a higher rate of speed.

One problem with these chutes is that they have a tendency to be unstable in windy conditions. Therefore, it is most effective to have the athlete run into the wind, although this is not always practical unless there is enough space available. The chute is most effective in still air or indoors. The chutes can be used with a group of 10-12 athletes if the workouts are well organized. I have also used chutes in rehab to reinforce correct (i.e., aligned hips, straight spine) posture and increase the athlete's proprioception when the chute is moving side to side. If adequate space is available, the chute works well for lateral speed and agility work such as planting and cutting and backpedaling.

The harness uses the resisted method of training and serves as a great teaching tool for developing sprint mechanics. It consists of a rope or cord attached to the athlete by a harness or belt with multiple hooks and is especially effective for working on the start and acceleration phase. When using this tool, it is best if a coach provides the resistance so that the proper amount is consistently applied.

Sometimes, there is a tendency for the holder to provide excessive resistance, which slows down the movement too much. This need for a holder limits the use of the harness with large groups of athletes.

There are a number of different types of harnesses from which to choose, and I have found that the best harnesses place the resistance as close as possible to the athlete's center of gravity. It is also helpful for the harness to have multiple attachment hooks for the resistance, so that it can be used for lateral speed and agility training and for it to possess the ability to release the resistance in order to create a contrast situation. I have not had good experiences with the shoulder type of harness, which attaches over both arms in a figure-eight pattern, as the athletes feel that the shoulder straps pull the torso back too much and interfere with arm action.

Tubing towing devices use a heavy grade of surgical tubing attached to the athlete with a belt and work in the opposite manner of the harness. They utilize the assisted method of training to create a running velocity that is greater than what can be achieved under normal conditions. They can also be used for resistance, although they are not as effective in this capacity because the resistance increases with the distance of the run.

The major drawback to tubing is that it does not provide a lot of control. It creates a much faster acceleration—almost a jerk—from the start, as opposed to a steady, even pull, making it effective primarily for shorter distances of 20 to 30 yards. There is also a definite safety risk factor of getting the rubber tubing out of the way when slowing down. Therefore, these devices should not be used by a large group unless there is a sufficient space available.

Pulley towing devices utilize both the assisted and resisted method of training. They work like tubing towing devices but are controlled by the puller instead of the tubing. In my experience, this tool offers the smoothest, most natural form of resistance and assistance. It does, however, require more skill on the part of the tower, as there is a different feel for each athlete. Therefore, it is best for the puller to be a coach or someone experienced to pull. It is important to remember that only a small increase in speed is desired and not to pull so hard that the athlete gets out of control. Another plus to this device is that it is much safer to use than others because a release in tension is all it takes to release the towing rope. This tool can be used in a group only when there are enough experienced people available to provide the towing or the resistance.

Sleds use the resisted method of training, as they attach to the athlete with a clip and a rope and work to improve an athlete's acceleration. They offer the ability to quantify the load as one can vary the amount of resistance added to the sled. (Remember the 10-Percent Rule, however: do not load the sled so heavily that it significantly slows the action.)

With these tools, it is important that the rope attaching the sled to the athlete is of adequate length so that when the athlete stops, the sled does not continue to slide and hit the back of the athlete's legs. Some sleds actually roll on wheels, but I have found them less effective because they rely on heavier external loading for resistance rather than a combination of resistance from external loading and the friction of sliding. They are also not as safe because they continue to roll after the athlete stops.

The 10% rule is the guide for both resistance and assistance training.

Weighted pants consist of tight fitting pants with pockets to hold weights. They offer the resisted method of training, developing specific strength by applying a weighted load directly to the legs. The proximal resistance of this device provides less interference with natural running mechanics than some of the aforementioned tools.

For the pants to work effectively, it is important that they fit very snugly so that there is no bounce or movement of the weights. Another key is adding the correct amount of weight. This tool has good rehab applications and works well with lateral speed and agility drills because of the specific resistance.

These pants currently are manufactured in three different types of materials. Neoprene shorts fit very snugly but can be very hot. Lycra can also provide a tight fit and has more breathability. Cotton or mixtures do not always offer the tight fit and thus are more difficult to determine the proper size.

Like the weighted pants, the weight vest uses the resisted method of training to develop specific strength. It is effective because it provides resistance close to the center of mass (i.e., the torso) and thus does not interfere with the movement patterns. Also like the weighted pants, a snug fit is important so that the weight seems part of the athlete.

Elevated shoes look like normal sneakers except that they are elevated in the front, under the ball of the foot. They help develop specific strength in the lower leg and use the resisted method. From my view, they are most effective for skipping exercises, jump rope, sprint drills, and lateral speed and agility drills. However, I have not found them advantageous for development of straight ahead speed; the weight of the shoe can cause the foreleg to swing out prematurely, which creates a tendency to overstride. These shoes now come in two models: with cleats for use on grass and turf, which makes them much safer, and with a flat sole for use indoors where there is better footing.

Stick ladders consist of a series of wooden or plastic dowels placed at sequential increments and attached by a nylon cord. The ladder is placed on the ground and the athlete must step into each of the open spaces. This serves to teach the mechanics of acceleration and help to develop efficiency of movement. By teaching proper stride position, the distribution of effort in acceleration is reinforced. It is also easy to use the ladder for lateral speed and agility work.

Be careful not to overuse this tool, however, because it can result in a high-frequency, low-power, output acceleration pattern. Also, make sure the ladders are adjustable to accommodate different stride patterns.

Rubber bands are placed around the athlete's ankles and use the resisted method to develop specific strength in the abductors and adductors of the hip. These muscles are especially important in improving lateral speed and agility, and in preventing and rehabilitating injuries. The bands come in lengths ranging from 8 to 24 inches, while the most effective width for many different strength levels is the one and one-half-inch band. These tools are inexpensive, safe, and easy to use by either individuals or a large group.

The slide board utilizes the resisted method of training for the development of lateral speed and agility and specific leg strength. It consists of a slippery board on which the athlete moves back and forth. It is important that the board can be adjusted to accommodate different leg lengths and different training objectives. I have found wider boards to be more useful because they allow the athletes to slide at an angle. A sturdy, angled step-board is also essential if the board is going to be used for speed development.

There is not just one product or training method for speed development that is significantly better than all the others. What is most important is that the coach knows how each product can be used relative to the strengths and weaknesses of the individual athlete and the objectives of the training ◆

At the End Of Your Endurance

When people think of endurance they usually associate it with such sports as running, swimming, cycling, and crew. But the steady requirements of these activities comprise only one type of endurance — one which does not reflect the endurance demands of the majority of team sports.

Simply stated, endurance is the capacity to resist fatigue. So, a player in a transitional game like soccer will have different endurance needs than a marathoner, who has different endurance needs from a basketball player. It follows that the endurance training for each sport should reflect these differences.

With this in mind, we need to shift our thinking away from endurance as a long-duration aerobic activity and realize that the great majority of the sports that we train for are not continuous activities, but consist of short bursts of high-intensity work with short low-intensity breaks for recovery. They are mixed aerobic/anaerobic work or are often purely anaerobic.

Not just for long-distance runners, endurance training is crucial for any athlete — as long as it is sport specific.

Aerobic Endurance

Aerobic capacity, measured as VO_2 max, is the gold standard measurement of endurance. VO_2 max can be defined as the maximum amount of oxygen that your heart can pump to your muscles and that your muscles can use to produce energy. In absolute terms, it is expressed in liters per minute of oxygen consumed. In relative terms, it is expressed in milliliters of oxygen per kilogram of body weight (ml/kg). It is usually measured in a maximum effort test on the treadmill.

Each athlete's VO_2 max is ultimately determined by genetics, and research has shown that an individual's peak VO_2 max can be reached with training for up to 12 to 18 months. After that, it levels off and will not — improve significantly — even with large volumes of work. Once that peak level is reached, training should focus work at a high percentage of VO_2 max for longer periods of time.

Before you rush out and have your team scheduled for VO_2 max tests, however, let's look a little closer at its role in athletics. First of all, sports are not contests of who has the highest VO_2 max, they are contests of who can perform the best in the required arena. If VO_2 max was the prime determining performance factor, then Frank Shorter would not have won the 1972 Olympic marathon. In fact, he would not have even made the US team because his VO_2 max of 77 ml/kg is low for a world-class marathon runner. Instead, Shorter is a classic example of an individual who was very efficient, i.e., he was able to run at a high percentage of max without accumulating significant lactate buildup.

I am of the opinion that VO_2 max is significantly overrated as a measurement of endurance ability, especially for game sports. It has been utilized because it is relatively convenient and easy to measure, and there is a vast amount of research on it. But for the most part, too much time is spent on max VO_2 training for sports that do not require a high VO_2 max as a direct performance factor.

It would be more valuable to spend the time training to improve the endurance capacity specific to the demands of the sport rather than raising the level of general endurance. Simply put, endurance is more than VO_2 max and training the energy systems. According to Harre, "The level of endurance is determined first and foremost by the functional efficiency of the cardiovascular, metabolic, and nervous systems, as well as by the level of coordination of the activities of the organs and systems of the body."

Another pitfall of using VO_2 max is that it is dependent on heart rate, and in intermittent sprint games,

Figure One: Testing Endurance

Tests for endurance should reflect the endurance demands of the sport. They should be designed to challenge the athlete and give specific feedback to direct the endurance training so that the training time is optimized.

- Beep Test — This is a multi-stage shuttle test in which the athlete runs back and forth over a 20-meter distance at predetermined paces based on an auditory tone. It reflects the endurance demands of intermittent sports. It is also easily administered and can be used periodically throughout the season to assess fitness levels.
- Cooper Test — A continuous 12-minute for distance run on a track.
- Wingate Test — A test of anaerobic power done on a friction bike.
- Cunningham Test — A test of anaerobic capacity on a treadmill.
- 300-Yard Shuttle — A test of anaerobic capacity that can be done on a field, court, or track. The athlete runs 25 yards six times, down and back. Three or five minutes of recovery are allowed before a second run, depending on the sport. The score is the average time of the two runs.

Figure One: Six-Week Endurance Training Cycle

	Monday	Tuesday	Wednesday	Thursday	Friday	Saturday	Sunday
Week One	10x100@ 60% 30 sec rec	Circuit Training: 30 sec work 15 sec rec	Continuous 20 min	Recovery: Pool Workout	Fartlek: 15 min Recovery: Pool Workout	Circuit Training: 45 sec work 15 sec rec	Rest
Week Two	12x100@ 60% 30 sec rec	Circuit Training: 30 sec work 15 sec rec	Continuous 25 min	Recovery: Pool Workout	Fartlek: 20 min	Circuit Training: 45 sec work 15 sec rec	Rest
Week Three	2 (8x100)@ 60% 30 sec rec	Circuit Training: 30 sec work 15 sec rec	Continuous 25 min	Recovery: Pool Workout	Fartlek: 25 min	Circuit Training: 45 sec work 15 sec rec Recovery: Pool Workout	Rest
Week Four	10x30 sec @ 70% 30 sec jog rec	Circuit Training: 30 sec work 15 sec rec	Continuous 30 min	Recovery: Pool Workout	Fartlek: 15 min 10 min of 10 sec bursts	Circuit Training: 45 sec work 15 sec rec Recovery: Pool Workout	Rest
Week Five	12x30 sec @ 70% 30 sec jog rec	Circuit Training: 30 sec work 15 sec rec	Continuous 35 min	Recovery: Pool Workout	Fartlek: 15 min 12 min of 10 sec bursts	Circuit Training: 45 sec work 15 sec rec Recovery: Pool Workout	Rest
Week Six	10x30 sec @ 80% 45 sec jog rec	Circuit Training: 30 sec work 15 sec rec	Continuous 40 min	Recovery: Pool Workout	Fartlek: 20 min	Circuit Training: 45 sec work 15 sec rec Recovery: Pool Workout	Rest

there can be tremendous variation in heart rate throughout the course of the activity. The maximum heart rate of an athlete is also different for each activity — there is a heart rate maximum for swimming, for biking, and for running, and there is also a competition and practice maximum. So, which do you choose? Therein lies the problem.

A preferable alternative is to base endurance training on a percentage of the athlete's best at a specific test distance or time, or a percentage of maximum effort. While the latter is somewhat subjective, it can work quite well with coaches' input and feedback because a major part of endurance training is learning to be comfortable with a level of discomfort. I use terms like "easy," "medium," "hard," or "all out," to describe the quality of the effort relative to competition effort. (This is just a coaching adaptation of Borg's perceived exertion scale.)

Anaerobic Endurance

At the opposite end of the spectrum from VO_2 max is anaerobic work. However, in the context of endurance, to label something anaerobic is not accurate enough. It is important to make the distinction between alactate and lactate anaerobic work. In alactate anaerobic work there is no lactate accumulation. Alactate work is short-burst, high-intensity work that occurs in most games or, for example, the 100m in track, where the time frame is 12 seconds or less.

In lactate anaerobic work, there is a buildup of lactic

acid which, if continued, would force the athlete to stop the activity. This is what occurs in a 400m run in track. In most "game sports" there is seldom, if ever, any significant lactate buildup because the duration of the intense activity is not long enough. It usually takes 40 seconds or more of high-intensity activity to get significant lactate buildup.

Mechanical Efficiency

Beyond energy systems, mechanics also figure into endurance training. The buzzword for proper mechanics is "efficiency," which is used a lot in reference to endurance performance. It is not uncommon to hear comments like: "He looks really efficient."

What does that mean? I have always felt that efficiency is a convergence of physiological and biomechanical factors characterized by economy of effort. Ultimately, it is the ability to operate at a higher percentage of maximum without undue fatigue.

The biomechanics of movement are often overlooked as a factor in efficiency and efficiency is a hidden factor in optimizing training. For example, a basketball player who is asked to run for 30 to 40 minutes and has poor running mechanics will not be able to push hard enough to get a real endurance benefit from the workout. Therefore, good movement mechanics for the chosen activity are key to improving efficiency.

One more factor in the endurance equation is the effect of not training with sport specificity in mind. Improperly designed endurance training programs that do not reflect the demands of the sport and the qualities of the individual athlete can actually be detrimental to speed, power, and skill. According to Rushall and Pyke, "When an athlete trains in a predominantly aerobic fashion the enzymes for anaerobic energy production are reduced through lack of stimulation and the capacity for sustained sprinting deteriorates."

Into Practice

The obvious question then is: what do my athletes have to do to build up endurance for a sport such as basketball, soccer, football, or volleyball? The answer is relatively simple, with complex implications.

Essentially, the key is to design your endurance training program to meet the specific demands of the sport, the position or event, and the athletes' individual qualities. Since game sports are characterized by continuous changes of intensity and movement, this usually entails carefully sequencing the work and emphasizing a mix of interval, variation, and continuous aerobic work. Another objective in developing endurance for these types of activities is to teach and practice economy of movement.

The first step is to classify the differing types of endurance. I prefer the endurance classification delineated by Harre in his classic work "Principles of Sport Training."

Long Duration Endurance covers 11 minutes to several hours without a significant reduction in speed. The primary energy source is aerobic. It is broken down further as: Long Duration I: 11 minutes to 30 minutes; Long Duration II: 30 minutes to 90 minutes; Long Duration III: longer than 90 minutes.

Medium Duration Endurance covers 2 to 11 minutes in duration. The energy sources are mixed aerobic and anaerobic.

Short Duration Endurance covers 45 seconds to 2 minutes in duration. The primary energy source is anaerobic. It is related to levels of stored energy (phosphate), ability to tolerate lactic acid, and ability to utilize lactic acid.

Speed Endurance covers activities that last in the range of 10 to 60 seconds, with the primary objective being to minimize speed loss. The primary energy source is anaerobic.

Strength Endurance covers the ability to repeat strength oriented movements in a climate of fatigue. The primary energy source is anaerobic.

The second step is to understand endurance training methods. They can be broken down as follows:

Continuous: The activity is carried out continuously for a prescribed period of time, and there are no breaks. In continuous work, a methodological progression is to increase five minutes a day per week until your athlete is up to their target times. For example, a steady run used for recovery could be a continuous exercise. The run should be steady — not a slow, plodding jog — for 20 to 45 minutes. Use this no more than two times a week unless it is a warm-up or a cooldown run.

Changing: Changes occur in the intensity of the effort in a predetermined fashion. For example, in a 10-second burst, the athlete bursts hard with maximum effort for 10 seconds then slows down and coasts for 30 seconds, repeating this pattern for the total specified time (e.g., two sets of six min., finish with a 10-min. steady cooldown run).

Variation: Commonly called "Fartlek," which is the Swedish word for "speed play," these are unstructured changes in intensity of effort. Fartlek is used to simulate the demands of the game with quick starts and stops over longer periods of time. The work bouts should vary from as short as 15 seconds to as long as 90 seconds. The athlete should run with a hard effort; jog, walk, or skip for recovery; continue to alternate in this manner until the total time objective is completed. For example: 20 min. total time with 15 hard efforts dispersed throughout.

Interval Work — Definite programmed periods of work and recovery. The key to interval training is the manipulation of the rest interval between work bouts and the ability to hold the rest interval without compromising the quality of the work.

This is the main medium for producing specific training effects due to the ability to tailor the workout to suit individual needs. The emphasis should be on quality of work. It should be noted that in swimming, interval work generally is done with shorter rest periods because of the ability to recover more quickly due to 1) the horizontal position of the body, 2) body weight supported by the water, and 3) efficient removal of heat through the water.

Extensive Tempo Interval: Work that is less than 80 percent of the athlete's best time for a particular distance. I have also used 80-percent effort as a guide when the best time for a particular distance is not known. This is what is commonly called aerobic interval work. The goal is to bring the time of the run down with each cycle while still maintaining the prescribed rest interval. For example: three sets of 5 x 100 at 24 sec. (60-percent effort) with a 30-sec. rest between runs and 3 min. rest between sets. Another example would be: 10 x 30 sec. run, 30 sec. jog recovery.

Intensive Interval: 80 to 90 percent of best time for a particular distance or between 80 to 90 percent effort. Care must be taken to not do too much work in this range due to significant lactate buildup. For example: 10 x 30 sec. run at 80 percent effort, 1 min. jog recovery.

Repetition: As opposed to interval training, this type of work is characterized as complete a recovery as possible. For example: 3x 45 sec. runs (all out) with 12 to 15 min. recovery or 1 x 60-sec. run with 10 min. recovery, 1 x 45 sec. with 8 min. recovery, 1 x 30 sec.

Circuit Training: The primary method for training strength endurance. It consists of alternating various strength exercises for high repetitions (15 to 50 reps).
All of the above methods can be adapted to various modes of exercise, such as running, swimming, cycling, stairclimbing, slide board, rowing, cross-country skiing, or water workouts. It is important to take into consideration the differing energy costs of the various modes of work, as well as the weightbearing nature of the activity.

Organizing Endurance Training

So how do you use the above information to structure a workout sequence for the endurance demands of an intermittent sprint game like soccer or basketball? Figure One is an example of a six-week cycle of endurance training. Each week is set up with one interval workout, one fartlek workout, two circuit workouts, and one lower-intensity continuous aerobic workout per week. The aerobic workout is intended to be a recovery workout at a conversational pace. None of these workouts are designed to be excessively long in duration. Therefore, they must be done with intensity and concentration for maximum benefit.

The chosen mode of exercise is running, in which it is always important to emphasize good running mechanics. If you are plodding through the workouts, there is little or no carryover to the game and the risk of injury is greater. It is intended that these workouts be preceded by a thorough warm up and followed by a good cooldown. ◆

References
Harre, Dietrich, (ed.) *Principles of Sports Training: Introduction to the Theory and Methods of Training,* Berlin: Sportverlag, 1982.

Rushall, Brent S., and Pyke, Frank S., *Training for Sports and Fitness,* Melbourne: Macmillan Education Australia, PTY LTD 1990.

Leading the Pack

This chapter will concentrate on training for traditional endurance events — especially distance running. By definition, this will encompass events that last from three minutes to several hours in duration. These events are inherently continuous in nature, as opposed to the mostly intermittent nature of team sports. Even though this article is directed toward running, its ideas are applicable to other endurance activities, such as cycling, swimming, cross country skiing, and rowing. Many of the technical considerations I discuss are different, but the general training philosophies are the same.

Rather than rehash conventional wisdom readily available through a variety of sources, I will center my thoughts on observations and first-hand experience gleaned from training runners for distances from the 800 meters to the marathon. I must emphasize that the focus here is on training to race — training to run fast is the essence of endurance training. Somewhere along the way, many people got the mistaken impression that endurance training is about the runner's high and that it should be some sort of pleasurable, Zen-like, meditative experience. Training to run fast for prolonged periods of time demands hard, directed work that is concentrated and planned. Sometimes, it is very uncomfortable.

One of my motivations for writing this is the lack of success in American middle distance and distance runners over the past 20 years, especially on the male side of the ledger. There are many reasons for this, not the least of which is an increasing sedentary lifestyle among our young people, as well as an overabundance of overprocessed foods and an overprescription of antibiotics (which many people believe contribute to our high rates of asthma). In my opinion, perhaps the biggest reason has been a lack of proper training.

There is little that is new in the preparation of endurance athletes. But, sometimes we have to look back in order to move ahead. Methods like strength training, core training, resistance running, and recovery were all ingredients in the regimens of former American distance running champions. I would like to review some of the methods that worked in the past, which we now better understand because of applied sport science research, as discussion points for where we need to go in the future to better prepare endurance runners and, for that matter, endurance athletes in general.

Training Systems

A systematic approach is the key to successful endurance training. A central element of any good system is time. It takes time to develop all the capacities necessary for success in distance running. Bill Bowerman, the late, great coach from the University of Oregon, is a great example of a coach who had a system with the big picture in mind. He knew that it would take time for his runners to mature. His program was very progressive in that each runner's mileage and overall workload were very controlled so that he or she could handle the workload. His hard/easy principles stressed the importance of recovery. He understood that the body needed time to recover from hard training efforts, so he scheduled easy days to allow for adaptation. His system was an eclectic one that borrowed from other systems he studied and adapted to the American environment and the developing collegiate athlete.

> *Speed must be worked on first and foremost, and it must be part of every training cycle. Speed-development work can be as simple as sprint drills, light acceleration drills, or simply finishing each run with eight to ten 100-meter fast strides.*

Arthur Lydiard, the famous distance coach from New Zealand, was known for the marathon phase of training. No doubt this base phase of his training was important, but I have always felt that the most important phase of his program was the hill-training phase. This was where his runners developed the specific strength for the powerful strides that led to the ability to handle a fast pace and also deliver a punishing finishing kick. He did not believe in weight training, but this hill phase accomplished the same purpose. Interestingly, his system produced top-ranked runners from the 800 meters to the marathon with athletes who had a wide variety of natural talent. This versatility is the true measure of an endurance-training system.

Percy Cerutty, the eccentric Australian coach, developed a system that put a heavy emphasis on the natural aspects of running. It incorporated a lot of resistance running in sand dunes and running barefoot, as well as a large emphasis on lifting relatively heavy weights. In many respects, Cerutty was ahead of his time in that his emphasis was on power as well as endurance. Franz Stampfl, in Australia, and Mihaly Igloi, in Hungary and later the United States, both had systems that depended heavily on interval training. This is a very efficient system of training that was first researched and perfected in Germany in the 1930s. Stampfl coached Roger Bannister to the first sub-four minute mile. It is interesting to note that Bannister, because of his medical school demands, only had one hour a day to train. That is one of the advantages of interval training: with limited time, it is possible to prepare for the intensity of the demands of racing.

Joe Vigil is an American coach who formerly coached at Adams State College in Colorado. He continues to coach post-collegiate runners today. His is a very eclectic system based on high-altitude training, which reflects his background as an exercise physiologist. Like most of the other great coaches who developed personalized training systems, he has evolved his methods based on his environment, incorporating hills and sand dunes as well as sustained hard-effort runs that climb 5,000 feet in altitude.

Speed First

Speed must be worked on first and foremost, and it must be part of every training cycle. I find it amusing when I hear runners say, "I have been doing base work, but I have not started speed work yet." These runners are not training to run fast; they are training to run far, and they hope that the speed will come. The inevitable result is undue soreness and greater risk of injury because of the abrupt change in the training program when they do start to run fast.

The key is to never get too far away from running fast. It should be part of the first training cycle of the year and of each subsequent training cycle. Speed-development work can be as simple as sprint drills, light acceleration drills, or simply finishing each run with eight to ten 100-meter fast strides. It may be a coaching cliché, but the winner of the race is the person who slows down the least. Therefore, the goal in training is to continually strive to run longer at a higher percentage of peak velocity. Rather than focusing on pace, it is better to focus on distribution of effort. Races, at any level, are seldom run at the physiological ideal of even pace. The goal is to distribute the effort as efficiently as possible over the entire race distance. It is interesting to note that the highly successful Moroccan school of distance running clearly acknowledges the importance of speed and power in distance running performance through their talent-identification test. They test a short sprint from a standing start, a middle distance race, and the standing long jump.

Running Mechanics

Running mechanics are a key aspect of running performance. It seems like everyone pays close attention to correct mechanics up to the 400 meters, but beyond that distance, it is as if it does not matter anymore, when, in fact, it actually could be just as important. Good, sound running mechanics can go a long way toward preventing injuries and optimizing stride length and rate for more efficient utilization of energy stores.

Improving running mechanics involves specific strengthening of the postural muscles as well as the legs. Technique practice in the form of drills should be part of daily training no matter what distance is being trained. Constant awareness of good running mechanics must be stressed during each run. What do good running mechanics consist of? It starts with good posture — erect carriage of the trunk. This is followed by good arm action — the arm carriage should be low so as not to cause undue fatigue. The shorter the race, the greater the amplitude of the arm action. The leg action should be short and controlled. High knee lift and excessively long strides are not rewarded. Efficiency is the end result of good distribution of effort and sound running mechanics.

Strength Training

The objective of strength training for the distance runner is the same as for any athlete: to strengthen the areas that are necessary to improve performance and prevent injury. Somehow, the mistaken notion has developed over the years that it is not necessary for the distance runner to strengthen the legs. Nothing could be further from the truth. The legs are the main propulsive mechanism in running. Therefore, a good multi-joint leg program will significantly help performance and prevent injury by better preparing the body for the forces incurred, particularly on landing. The key is to avoid hypertrophy methods. Undue mass can hinder performance (distance runners don't need huge arm, or even leg, muscles). That is simply addressed by using more sets and keeping the reps low and the weight relatively heavy (relative to the athlete's weight and training needs). Bodyweight exercises and circuit training are particularly effective modes of strength training.

Somehow, the mistaken notion has developed over the years that it is not necessary for the distance runner to strengthen the legs. Nothing could be further from the truth.

Conventional wisdom advises against the distance runner using plyometric training. To a certain extent, that is true, but it is more the form of plyometrics than plyometric training itself. While super-high-intensity plyos, like depth jumps and box jumps, can be counterproductive for the 800-meter and 1500-meter runner and the steeplechaser, plyos in the form of hops and bounds at very low volume and used in conjunction with strength training, are very important. For the longer events, simple skipping (jumping rope) and sprint drills will have a plyometric effect, which will have a positive carryover to the dynamics of the stride.

Neural vs Metabolic

In order to improve distance running performance, it is necessary to think beyond the heart and lungs. It is a given that to be a successful distance runner, it is necessary to have a highly developed and efficient cardiovascular system as evidenced by a high max VO_2. Max VO_2 is only one piece of the puzzle, however. We now know that once a runner has trained his or her VO_2 to a high level, there is little room for improvement. VO_2 maximum can only be improved to a certain extent; after that, the improvement and adaptation probably take place in the active muscles. Fortunately, it is relatively easy to maintain the VO_2 at that high level.

Along with this, it has become quite popular to focus on training the energy systems. It is important to remember, however, that the energy systems are intensity-dependent, not time-dependent. If I walk across a room, I am using my body's aerobic energy system, while if I sprint across the room, I am utilizing my anaerobic energy system. Either way, the body must produce ATP in order for muscle action to occur, and ATP can be manufactured both through aerobic and anaerobic means. It is intensity of effort, not duration, that is most important in training.

Perhaps we need to focus more on the neural aspect of endurance performance. Running fast for prolonged periods of time demands a high level of coordination of all systems of the body. This should make us more aware of training the nervous system; it is the nervous system that commands and controls the body. The muscles are slaves of the brain.

LSD

"Long, slow distance" is a term originally coined to describe running at a steady pace to develop an aerobic base. Unfortunately, as it evolved, the emphasis was on SLOW. This was a huge mistake. The result was proficiency at running slowly for a prolonged period. This has little carryover to racing — remember, the goal of training is to prepare to race. The emphasis in this method should be on long, STEADY distance. Select a degree of effort that allows the runner to run a steady effort for the duration of the distance with good running mechanics. This type of training needs to be a means to an end and must be combined with other means of training, including speed work. Unfortunately, for many runners, it has become an end to itself.

The Finest Interval

Interval training is one of the key foundations for race preparation. Four variables can be manipulated in interval training: distance, number of repetitions, rest interval, and intensity (represented by the time of the rest interval). It has been my experience that the key to effective interval training is to focus on rest. To harden the athlete to the stress of racing, multiple sets with shorter rest intervals are the best way to prepare. This is perhaps the biggest change in interval training over the years. Mihaly Igloi, who built his training system on interval training, based the intensity of the interval on the following descriptors of the progressive gradations leading up to race effort:

- Easy — used for recovery
- Medium easy — moderate effort
- Medium — a little harder, but still conversational
- Swing — fast, but still controlled (you should still feel like you have another gear)
- Fast — just as the name implies
- Race — highest effort

These descriptors are nothing more than a perceived exertion scale. The Borg Scale, used extensively in exercise testing and cardiac rehabilitation, scientifically validates the concept of this scale. This is a method to get the runner to tune into his or her body and feel the effort required by the particular interval. I have found this to be an especially effective system.

Recovery & Regeneration

As I mentioned earlier, the hard/easy method was a cornerstone of the Bowerman method. What this simply tells us is that we must be cognizant of recovery as a key to training. It is during recovery that the training adaptations occur. It is important to carefully plan recovery days as well as recovery cycles into the overall training plan. Further, recovery does not simply mean sitting around — external means of recovery, such as hot and cold contrast showers or baths, sauna, and massage, should be a regularly scheduled part of the training plan. Hydration is perhaps one of the most important aspects of recovery.

Periodization

Periodization relates to the timing of the application of the training stimulus. It is, in essence, balancing all components of training relative to the individual needs of each runner. It is helpful to break the training into manageable time periods that allow for specific adaptation to the imposed demands of that respective training period. Because of the nature of running, I have found it easier to point toward a definite peak in performance. I have found that once a runner achieves a peak, it's possible to remain at a fairly high percentage of that peak for six to eight weeks depending on the athlete's training age.

The key to effective interval training is to focus on rest. To harden the athlete to the stress of racing, multiple sets with shorter rest intervals are the best way to prepare.

Usually, a race is seen as the event to peak for. In this scenario, it is imperative to carefully plan the racing schedule to allow enough time to recover from the races and to properly prepare between races. It is also important to prepare for the demands of the championship meet by simulated trials and finals on back-to-back days. It is better to see how the athlete adapts to this type of stress by simulating the competition in a controlled training situation.

Beware, however, that over-racing is one cause of overtraining. I believe that racing not only taxes the runner's physiological reserves, but also severely taxes the psychological reserves. The runner must look forward to racing in order to be an effective racer.

In order to make periodization work, it is necessary to put more of an emphasis on monitoring training. Monitoring can be as simple as maintaining a detailed training log or as complicated and scientific as blood testing and ongoing heart-rate monitoring (which are not available to most people). A simple fatigue index that rates the runner's subjective feeling of effort and fatigue on a 10-point scale following a workout is particularly effective. Simply asking an athlete how hard a training session was to him or her is in some ways more effective than invasive methods.

Cross Training

Cross training is when an athlete undertakes training in a discipline other than his or her main sport for the sole purpose of enhancing performance in his or her primary event. It has been my experience that those athletes who utilize cross training the most are those who already have a tendency to chronically overwork and are looking for another way to punish themselves. I feel that this is another training myth that has actually detracted from sound training. It certainly has very little foundation in sports science research. For a runner to get in the pool for anything more than a recovery session is time ill spent. The same is true for biking.

Time would be better spent strength training or working on flexibility, both areas that tend to be ignored. Most of the time, they are ignored because the runner feels he or she does not have enough time to fit them in. Yet those same runners can find the time to swim for thirty minutes or bike for an hour. It is all a matter of priorities. Cross training may be okay for the recreational athlete seeking to relieve the boredom of training, but for the high-level athlete it is virtually useless.

Remember, the purpose of the plan is to prepare the runner to run fast over his or her chosen distance. Building a training program from the above elements — speed, good running mechanics, and strength training with a focus on intensity and optimal recovery in a well-thought-out, periodized yearly plan — is guaranteed to deliver results for any endurance athlete. ◆

Rethinking Periodization

Classic periodization is a concept that is very appealing in theory, but is not very practical for contemporary sports. Periodization originated in the former Soviet Union, where all aspects of athletes' lives were controlled. This control included diet, lifestyle, the athletes' competitive schedules, and even controlled doping. This systematic doping program has been extensively documented in two books: *Doping In Sport* (Doping Dokumente: von der Forschung zum Betrug), by Brigitte Berendonk and Faust's Gold; and *Inside the East German Doping Machine*, by Steven Ungerleider.

When total control and systematic doping are removed from the equation, periodization is simply planning, organizing, and monitoring your training into a structure that develops all biomotor qualities in a sequential and progressive manner. This structure made periodization work in the past, and it can make periodization work in your program today. The big question is, how can that be achieved without the use of 24-hour control and the drugs that were applied in classic periodization?

The answer is to shrink the long-term time frame of classic periodization into much shorter, controllable periods of time. This adaptation of the periodization concept is something that I call "Planned Performance Training," or PPT.

Implementing PPT

Begin the process of creating a PPT program for your athletes by carefully determining what the finished product should be. This finished product is a measurable performance goal such as a longer jump or a faster sprint time.

Next, you need to create a "year plan." The goal of this year plan is to attain the finished product that we've just defined. When I talk about a year, I refer to a "training year," which can be a July-to-July program for a basketball athlete, an academic year for a high school athlete, and so on. The year plan should contain all details that can affect your athlete's training goals, such as the initial condition of your athlete, the length of the competitive season, overlapping seasons, when competition begins, when vacations occur, and even when academic exams are scheduled.

Once this year plan is completed, you can fill in the elements of that plan. Working backwards from the desired goal, divide the year plan into blocks. Each block has one or more general themes, such as speed, strength, or endurance. The themes could also include a major and minor emphasis on training. For example, a block can have a major emphasis on speed and a minor emphasis on strength training.

How long should the block be? The time frame for each block is determined by the time it takes for the athlete to reach the defined conditioning goals. In my experience, the time frame for blocks averages about four weeks, but some go as short as two weeks for an introductory teaching block to as long as six weeks for a general preparation block.

To work properly, one block must flow into another without apparent, abrupt changes. Placement and timing of blocks should also be interchangeable to allow for varied rates of progress. The following are basic examples of the types of blocks that I have used in my training programs:

Introductory Block — This consists of short periods of time to introduce new methods, skills, or tactics. The goal here is teaching, not training. This block can be as short as seven days or as long as fourteen days, depending on the athlete's level of development.

Preparatory Block — There is no competition during this block. The emphasis is to raise work capacity or to address specific technical deficiencies. This block can have a very general emphasis for a developing athlete or a very narrow, specific emphasis for an elite athlete.

Competition I Block — The goal during this block is adapting the work done in a preceding preparatory block to a competitive mode. Even though the athlete is competing this is subservient to the training.

Competition II Block — This encompasses the all-important competitions. The goal during this block is application-type work, which refines what was done in the Competition I block.

Transition Block — This is an active block that allows no detraining. The goals are to regenerate, rehabilitate, and remediate (to address any fundamental deficiencies). During the season, this type of block will probably never be more than three days in duration. Between competitive seasons, it is ideal if this block is one month in duration.

Table One shows how this generalized block concept is applied to a specific sport, which in this case is a year-long block program that I designed for elite high school soccer players.

The Sessions

Next, you need to plan the training sessions that make

> *Classic periodization is a concept that has outlived its usefulness in light of the demands of the contemporary competitive schedule.*

 The Gambetta Method

Table One: Block Program for High School Soccer

Block One. Pre-season (August)

Major emphasis:
Speed/acceleration (short)
LSA
   Footwork
   Change of direction
Strength
   Body weight
   Plyometrics
   Core
Endurance I (extensive tempo)
Skill

Minor emphasis:
Endurance II (intensive tempo)
Speed endurance
Testing
Recovery

Block Two. Fall Club Season

Major emphasis:
Speed/acceleration (long)
LSA
   Footwork
   Change of direction
   Obstacle avoidance
Strength
   Weight training
   Core — multi throws
   Plyometrics
Speed endurance (ASSE)
Endurance II (intensive tempo)
Skill
Competition
Recovery

Minor emphasis:
Strength (body weight)
Endurance I (extensive tempo)
Speed (maximum)
Testing

Block Three. High School Season

Major emphasis:
Speed/acceleration
LSA
   Footwork
   Change of direction
Strength
   Body weight
   Core
Speed endurance
Skill
Competition
Recovery

Minor emphasis:
Strength (weight training)
Endurance I (extensive tempo)
Speed (maximum)
Testing

Block Four. Transition to spring club season

Major emphasis:
LSA
   Footwork
   Change of direction
   Obstacle avoidance
   Strength
   Testing
   Weight training
   Core
   Plyometrics
Speed endurance
Endurance II (intensive tempo)
Competition
Recovery

Minor emphasis:
Strength (body weight)
Speed/acceleration
Speed (maximum)
Endurance I (extensive tempo)

Block Five. Spring Club Season

Major emphasis:
Speed/acceleration
LSA
   Footwork
   Change of direction
   Obstacle avoidance
Strength
   Body weight
   Core
   Plyometrics
Speed endurance (ASSE)
Skill
Competition
Recovery

Minor emphasis:
Strength (weight training)
Endurance I (extensive tempo)
Speed (maximum)
Testing

up each block. When you plan these sessions, keep three considerations in mind.

First, in order to effectively construct training sessions, it is important to understand the physiological, biomechanical, and psychological changes that occur with training. Those changes are:

Immediate: What occurs during training and immediately after training.
Residual: The changes that occur from several hours to several days after a session.
Cumulative: This is the summation of training. The cumulative effect reflects long-term adaptation. It is the ultimate goal of your year plan — also called your "end product." Therefore, the focus of your session planning should be on the cumulative training effect.

Second, to achieve positive training results, carefully look at all of the components that make up each session. Be sure to emphasize complementary compo-

Table Two: Soccer Speed Acceleration Modules

Speed/Acceleration I
Soccer start
Balance start
Rollover start
Running start
Offset start
Crossover step
Running start with 360
Feint & go
Dancing start

Speed/Acceleration II
Curved sprint
Zig-zag sprint
Two-man weave
Partner opposite
Partner same

Speed/Acceleration III (with the ball & partner)
Ball drop reaction sprint
    a) one ball
    b) two balls
    c) face away
One touch & go, five meters
One touch & go, 10 meters
One touch & go, quick cut

To illustrate how modules should be arranged, the following are examples of speed/acceleration modules that I use for soccer players:

Monitor Progress

The plan should be accompanied by careful monitoring of the training to ensure that the desired adaptive response is achieved. Evaluating and monitoring training is a constant, ongoing process that should be part of each training session. Monitoring enables you to fine-tune the plan and the training according to the athlete's progress. It also helps you to better understand the effect of each training session and the effect on subsequent sessions. Monitoring the training should be approached from both subjective and objective perspectives.

Subjective monitoring includes a training demand rating scale, the ratio of sessions to hours trained, and video/qualitative analysis.

The training demand rating *scale* is a rating of perceived exertion, where the athlete rates the stress of that particular training session from one to ten. A one is very low stress and a ten is very high stress.

Ratio of number of training sessions to hours trained will vary depending on the sport, but over the years I have found that training is most effective when there are more sessions relative to hours trained, although this can differ for endurance sports such as cycling or swimming.

Video/qualitative analysis consists of subjectively viewing a video of the athlete in action for any obvious technical flaws.

Objective monitoring includes tests that can actually be measured. The tests include jump and throw, lab analysis, heart rates, biomechanical analysis, and competition evaluation.

Jump and throw test(s) will give a window into the athlete's nervous system by measuring the distance an athlete jumps or throws an object.

Blood & urine analysis/lab analysis gives an accurate reading into an athlete's actual physiological response and adaptation to training.

nents—ones that work together to enhance each other—both within and between sessions. For example, don't mix speed and endurance. Instead, mix speed and strength. Here are examples of complementary training units: speed and strength; strength and elastic strength; endurance and strength endurance; and skill, speed and elastic strength. Ultimately, the training sessions have more than a complementary relationship. They should enhance each other and mesh in an ultimately synergistic effect.

Third, you need to arrange the daily sessions into seven to 14-day cycles that are based on the athlete's ability to adapt to the training and then recover. When you create this cyclical structure, remember that the ability to recover varies from athlete to athlete. For example, I have one soccer athlete who can only tolerate one plyometric session in a seven-day cycle, while on the same team, I have another athlete who can tolerate three sessions in a seven-day training cycle.

Modules

Your next step is creating the modules that make up each session. The training module consists of specific combinations and sequences of exercises that are carefully selected to sequence and flow from one exercise to the next within the module.

Contemporary Challenges

Adapting periodization to your current sports program involves more than removing the use of drugs and total, long-term control of the athlete. There are also definite contemporary challenges that you'll need to consider, including the following:

- The decline of basic physical fitness levels and fundamental movement skills at the developmental level. This is the base of the pyramid and in my opinion, it has been weakened for two reasons. First, there is no more mandatory K-12 physical education in the United States, except in one state — Illinois. Second, our athletes are specializing at a younger age without an adequate base of general fitness and fundamental movement skills. This has a profound negative effect on the planning process.
- The demands of the extended competitive schedule. In many sports there are lengthy competitive seasons with no clearly defined off-seasons. This is characteristic from the developmental level through to the elite athlete. This makes traditional periodization difficult due to conflicting goals for different sports seasons.
- Drug influence/bias in traditional periodization models. As I previously stated, this has a profound effect on the planning process. Drugs that were used in traditional periodization significantly enhanced the athlete's ability to recover and handle heavier workloads. Those drugs are banned in virtually all contemporary sports programs due to their inherent dangers. However, without drugs there is almost no margin of error, which necessitates religious monitoring of the daily sessions to ensure your athletes are not being overworked.

Heart rate measurements should be taken before, during, and after the workout. Remember that there are many artefacts when using heart rate measurements. Be sure to consider each case individually.

Video/quantitative analysis using biomechanical analysis software is used to measure angular changes and velocities of an athlete in action. (For more information about video sports analysis and biomechanical software, log on to <www.AthleticSearch.com> and look for "Biomechanical Software" in the Bonus Editorial section.)

Competition evaluation. Never lose sight of the fact that the ultimate test is the competition itself. Carefully analyze each of the competition results relative to the plan and adjust the plan accordingly.

Remember, failing to plan is planning to fail. This is especially true with periodization. Take these ideas and adapt them to your situation. I feel confident that these ideas will help make planning and implementation of your training programs more effective. ◆

A Plan Behind the Dream

Failing to plan is planning to fail. In training an athlete, nothing could be more true. Above all else, planning is the most essential aspect of achieving athletic excellence.

In the United States, where we tend to think only in the terms of the present, the athlete development plan is a relatively foreign concept. However, the competitive reality of sports today demands that we do a better job of developing our talent. Our approach has been Darwinian — we have depended on numbers and only the strong have excelled. Those that have succeeded, in most instances, happened to be very good.

Over the years, I have had the opportunity to observe firsthand the development plans of several nations that do not have the benefit of large populations. They have to maximize the talent that is available. Needless to say, it is impressive to see how these countries develop their athletic talent to the fullest.

In this chapter my goal is to stimulate coaches to reorient their approach to developing athletes. Rather than survival of the few, I feel we need to incorporate a long-term, balanced approach that encompasses all levels of sport development. In youth sports, we must foster a better sense of what our goals are. And, in Olympic sports, we must do a much better job of identifying and nurturing our talent.

I am not advocating that we ask ten-year olds to leave their families and train 12 hours a day at a special sports center. What I am suggesting is that we must implement similar basic theories and goals at all levels of athletic development. The basis of a well-formatted plan should encompass the whole spectrum of athletic development — from child to champion.

Goals and Theories

There are three goals that all athlete development programs should share:

1. To provide a context for continuity and direction in the development of the athlete from entry level in the sport to retirement and preparation for life beyond sport.
2. To get a total commitment from all involved to support all levels of sport, recognizing that many people have a hand in the development of the athlete from the earliest exposure to the highest level of the respective sport.
3. To provide a positive experience to the entry-level athlete, realizing that only a small percentage of athletes will compete beyond that level, but that these athletes are potential officials, coaches, or at the very least, educated spectators and parents of future athletes. Beyond the basic goals, coaches must also share an adherence to certain theories of training. Here are my suggestions:

Developing talented athletes requires a long-term, balanced, systematic approach encompassing all levels of sport.

- A sound development plan must incorporate this fundamental progression at all levels and from level to level:
  Basic Conditioning
  Basic Skill
  Specific Advanced Conditioning
  Specific Advanced Skill

- The athlete must be an active participant in all aspects of the development process. Athlete development is not something that is done to the athlete, it is something that is done with the athlete.
- The concept of the "24-Hour Athlete" must be constantly stressed. The athlete can only train a fraction of the day, but what he or she does during those other hours is very important. Athletes must have their whole life in perspective to be successful in their chosen sport, and sport must improve their quality of life. Success in sport cannot be achieved without success in life.
- Ethics, character development, and accepted societal behavior must be stressed at each level of development. Athletes should be positive role models, and they must understand this role.
- The system must be coach driven. It is the coach who is in daily contact with the athlete, who knows the athlete best, and is best prepared to meet the athlete's needs. Therefore, educated coaches who understand their role in the total development process are the cornerstone of an athlete development plan.
- Talent identification and talent direction are essential. Talent direction, in fact, may be more important than identification. Just because an athlete is not successful at one sport does not mean that he or she will not be successful in another sport. Someone who tries basketball and is unsuccessful may be a good team handball player, but they will never know if they are not directed there.

A notable example is Alberto Juantorena of Cuba, double gold medalist in the 400m and 800m in Montreal in 1976. He was a national-level basketball player with good speed and endurance who was directed to track and field because it was recognized that his potential for ultimate success was greater on the track than on the court.

A Model

The above goals and theories are only a first step.

The harder part is applying them to specific sports and different levels of play. Accomplishing this entails answering many questions about the sport, developmental factors, and talent identification. However, do keep in mind that it is not the sport that determines the training process, but the development of the youth.

As an example, I have chosen to give a general overview of a developmental model for soccer. Given that each situation is slightly different, I have formatted this as a series of questions to guide you in developing of your own specific plan. An individual sport is a little less complex, but most of the concerns and considerations would be the same.

General Concerns
When is it appropriate to begin formal soccer training? What constitutes formal training? How should athletes develop their capabilities to the fullest and achieve mastery. In what ways can we reconcile individual development with team development? At the entry level? At the developing level? At the emerging elite level? At the elite level. What is the appropriate training content and technical skill relative to the level of development? What should be emphasized? When should it be emphasized?

What are the pedagogical principles that apply? Every aspect of the development program must be based on sound pedagogical principles. Each person involved in the process should have a clear understanding of these principles and their application. They must also recognize that there are different styles and rates of learning that will affect mastery of concepts and techniques.

Developmental Factors
In talking about different developmental levels, the athlete's "age" can encompass several factors, all of which must be considered. Therefore, determine the following: What is the Intellectual/Cognitive Age? What is the Biological Age? What is the Chronological Age? What is the Training Age? There are often vast differences between each. In addition, gender differences must be accounted for, both in terms of maturation and work capacity.

Dr. Istvan Balyi (Balyi and Way, 1995) of Canada has developed a paradigm of three distinct periods of athletic development:
- "Training to Train" encompasses two levels: the three to four years of initiation (usually during the early school years) and the five to seven years of basic training (pre-pubescent and during puberty).
- "Training to Compete" consists of three to four years of build-up training (post-pubescent).
- "Training to Win" can last six to ten years (or more!) and entails systematic high-level training during adulthood.

This paradigm is an excellent context in which to view the whole process of athlete development. (See Figure One.)

According to Balyi (1996), there is another important stage that precedes these three stages: the FUNdamental stage. This stage serves to introduce the sport in a recreational environment. The game must be modified to teach motor stimulation and basic coordination. (One example is micro soccer, where the game is played on very small fields with a limited number of players.)

After reviewing Balyi's paradigm, the following questions must be asked:
- What are the means of achievement of all the above factors at each developmental level?
- How many athletes participate at each level? Who continues to participate? Who leaves the program? Why?
- How many practices a week should there be at each level? What should the distribution be of practice emphasis relative to age group and level of development in regard to: individual skill, team tactics, team strategy, conditioning, speed, strength, stamina, and suppleness?
- What is the ideal ratio of training to competition at each stage of development? (Recognize that the games are a motivating factor at the earlier stages of development.) What is the recommended number of training hours per week for each stage of development? What is the recommended number of training sessions per week for each stage of development?
- How many years does it take for a player to make a team at the following levels: National, State, Junior National, Senior National, Olympic, World Cup?
- What individual criteria are necessary to achieve the above goals? How are these determined? Who determines them?

Talent Identification Plan
The two best ways to identify talent are to test basic motor components of soccer and observe skill in a play environment with different combinations of players. Keep in mind that success at a younger age is not a guarantee of success later on.

This is a broad overview of an athlete development plan and will need refinement for each sport and each level of play. It may also seem like an insurmountable task, since our society currently places little emphasis on coaching education, and most athletes experience several different coaches throughout their careers. However, if we can start to at least have the same basic theories and goals at each level of development — and understand how each level works with the next — we can make noticeable gains in the future. ◆

Paradigm of Development

	Training To Train	Training To Compete	Training To Win
Developmental Stages	Initiation and basic training	Buildup training	Systematic high level training
Movement Skill Development	Introduce fundamental movement skills	Master fundamental movement skills as a key component of sport skill	Incorporate fundamental movement skills into training skills and drills
Growth and Development	Pre-pubescent and pubescent	Pubescent and post-pubescent	Physical maturity
Technical Model	Basic skill	Advanced skill	Specific advanced skill
Knowledge of Game	Rules and position	Individual and team tactics	Team strategy and game analysis
Sportsmanship	Respect for teammates and coaches	Respect for officials	Respect for fans
Teamwork and Interaction	Interaction with coach and teammates	Cooperation in pursuit of team goals	Leadership
Nutrition	Principles of sound training diet	Pre-competition and competition diet	Individual program
Conditioning	Basic conditioning	Advanced conditioning	Specific advanced conditioning
Recovery and Regeneration	Understand role of recovery	Use recovery methods	Develop individual recovery routine
Emotional Development	Emotional control	Controlling competitive anxiety	Competitive attitude
Work Habits	Establish training routine	Refine training routine	Specific individual routine
Mental Control/Rehab	Monitor growth and development, assess any postural or structural predisposition to injury	Treat and rehab any injuries, address any chronic injury situations	Treat and rehab any injuries
Psychological Preparation	Self image development and focus	Goal setting, relaxation and visualization	Individual mental game plan

References

Balyi, Istvan, personal conversation, 1996.

Balyi, Istvan, and Way, Richard, "Long-Term Planning of Athlete Development, The Training to Train Phase," *BC Coach*, Fall 1995 pp. 2-9.

Johnson, Carl, "Are We Really Going in the Right Direction?" *Athletics Coach*, Vol. 22 #1, March 1988. pp. 17-20.

Thumm, Hans-Peter, "The Importance of the Basic Training for the Development of Performance." *New Studies in Athletes*, Vol. 2, #1, March 1987. pp. 47-64.

All Season Training

Training year-round is no longer an option for athletes. Gone are the days of actually having an off-season and using the preseason to get in shape. Given the extended length of the competitive season in most sports and the higher caliber of competition, year-round training is a must, even for younger, developing athletes.

Year-round training offers many advantages, including more time to work on weaknesses, the opportunity to go into more depth with different physical qualities, and the ability to think year-to-year rather than just within a training season. But year-round training requires careful planning to avoid the dangers of overtraining or simply getting stuck in a rut — it does not mean doing the same thing, or even training in the same sport for 12 months. In order to get the most out of training year-round, it is necessary to use a comprehensive approach, so that the training plan is an extension of a sound athletic career development plan.

I will discuss the major topics to consider as you develop a year-round training program. At times, I will focus on the younger, developing athlete — that is, up to high school and early college. While this population is most likely to show large improvements with year-round training, these athletes are also the most at-risk for such things as injuries and overtraining. It is also important to note that the effects of training can be cumulative, particularly if the athlete is training year-round for several years. Therefore, the training and each individual's progress have to be constantly evaluated and re-evaluated.

Training Windows

In his book, *Children and Sports Training: How Your Future Champions Should Exercise to Be Healthy, Fit, and Happy* (Stadion Publishing: Island Pond, Vermont, 1996), Jozef Drabik introduced the concept of "sensitive periods" in growth and development. Essentially, these sensitive periods are windows of opportunity for the optimum development of biomotor capacities and skill acquisition.

According to Drabik, these periods are a very important consideration when creating a year-round training plan for the younger, developing athlete. As he explains, "These sensitive periods are periods in human life when the organs and systems that determine a given ability (balance, endurance, speed, or any other ability) are undergoing intensive development. It is then that they are most receptive to a training stimulus developing that ability."

When training becomes a year-round endeavor — as it is for more and more athletes — new periodization strategies must be devised based on each athlete's level, goals, and place in the year-round plan.

These periods are especially important for the pre-pubescent athlete, because these windows close as quickly as they open. This underscores the importance of getting these young athletes into a good year-round training program. A well-conceived year-round training program ensures that the athlete will be training no matter when his or her window of developmental opportunity opens. With the older, more mature athlete, these periods become optimal training times that are influenced by more than just growth and development—the cumulative effect of factors such as number of years played and number of injuries. As an athlete's number of training years increases, you are less likely to see large jumps in his or her abilities or skills.

For the female athlete, the windows of training opportunity open earlier, because of earlier maturation. Therefore, female athletes must specialize earlier. For girls, the most important component that will open these windows of training opportunity may relate to strength training. In fact, it is my observation that the female athlete who begins a sound, well-rounded strength-training program early on — at about ten to 12 years of age — has a distinct advantage over her peers who do not. This is evident in both a different body composition and a better training adaptation.

Training Components and Progression

Strength is the precursor to speed and power development as well as a key to injury prevention. For this reason, for both boys and girls, strength training is a unifying thread that ties all the other year-round training components together. It is the element of training that should appear in all phases of the yearly program, but in different proportions as well as in different forms.

For the younger, developing athlete, a good year-round training program should include participation in multiple sports. The consensus is that early specialization yields early stagnation and, conversely, general, multi-sport participation yields long-term career development. This is a key concept to ensure well-rounded development. The athlete is training year-round, but there is a large variation in stimuli. Multi-sport participation also has a positive influence on coordination, giving the athlete a rich repertoire of motor skills to draw from when specialization does occur. Of course, the exceptions to this are sports like gymnastics and figure skating, where it is necessary to begin specializing at an early age.

Ideally, the younger, developing athlete — regardless of athletic potential or promise — would begin athletic participation in sports that complement each other. By complementary, I mean that he or she participates in a secondary sport that has training elements and movement patterns that will enhance the athlete's primary sport activity. An example would be soccer as the primary sport with track sprinting or jumping as the complementary sport. Another example would be basketball as the primary sport and volleyball as the complementary sport.

For the sports to be complementary, many aspects of training for the two sports should be similar. As the athlete gets better in a particular sport, a logical progression would be to begin emphasizing that particular sport. The key is to choose a sport but not be locked into a position or an event within that sport. For example, the football player should play several positions, including both offense and defense. The next step would be to specialize in a position or an event. This should occur when the athlete has reached physical and emotional maturity.

The progression during a training year and during a career can be summarized as follows:

Basic Conditioning — This is more important with the younger, developing athlete. Its importance decreases as training age increases.

Basic Technical Model — For the younger athlete, this is another very important component of the training year. As the athlete matures and technique is mastered, this also assumes less importance.

Specific Advanced Conditioning — This is based on the level of basic conditioning and allows the training to both focus on specific demands and be more rigorous. Taking weight training as an example, there is now a higher percentage of advanced plyometrics and more weights rather than medicine balls.

Advanced Technical Model — This is based on the basic technical model. The athlete is now able to perform more complex movements and combinations and work on advanced sport-specific technique.

The Goals
The goals of year-round training are very specific:
- In team sports, it is necessary to reconcile the needs of the individual player and the demands of the game with the needs of the team.
- Balance skill, technical, and tactical considerations with the physical demands of the game or sport.
- Train all components of athletic performance — the so-called "5S" approach — and allow for proper recovery/regeneration. (5S = skill, speed, stamina, strength, and suppleness.)
- Structure training weeks (microcycle) and training sessions for optimal results.

Strength training is a unifying thread that ties all the other training components together. It is the element of training that should appear in all phases of the yearly program, but in different proportions as well as in different forms.

- The constant that drives the system is competition. In order to accomplish these goals, one must control the ratio of training to competition. This is where the system tends to break down. Because of the length of the competitive schedule, there is seldom a defined off-season. In the community where I live, for example, baseball is a very popular youth sport. The high school season is anywhere from 25 to 32 games. The summer season can be as many as 40 games. Then there is a fall season where athletes can play an additional 25 games. This schedule is the same for an immature ninth grader or a very mature twelfth grader. When do the players train and prepare to play with such a schedule? This is the case for other sports as well. Basketball, volleyball, and soccer all have extended competitive seasons regardless of the age and stage of development of the athlete.

This is the crux of the problem: year-round competition without adequate time for year-round training. With an overemphasis on competition to the exclusion of training, development of the player is often a secondary consideration. It becomes a Darwinian process where the strong survive, although they do not always thrive. Those who are already good make it; those who could be good do not.

Thus, where possible, it is important to control the competition schedule within the year-round training schedule. There should be definite periods where the emphasis is on "training to train," with no competition or games scheduled. From an injury-prevention perspective, there must be planned breaks or unloading to allow for adaptation as well as maintain mental freshness. Psychological burnout is a distinct threat unless the program is structured to include breaks in the routine as well as variety in the training itself.

Vital Factors
As you develop a year-round training program, it's critical to consider the following factors to ensure an effective program that is well-suited to a particular athlete.

Developmental Level:
- At the initiation stages, it should not even be called training; it should be play with a loose structure.
- The developing athlete should begin year-round training, but with a multi-sport approach.
- The emerging athlete should begin specialization in a very structured, year-round program.

Biological/Chronological Development — Biological age must be considered over chronological age. There is a possibility of huge differences based on early or late maturation.

Intellectual/Cognitive Development — The athlete's

ability to process and understand information can be a big factor when he or she is participating in a sophisticated, year-round program.

Emotional Development — Emotional maturity is necessary to handle the ups and downs of training and competition.

Training Age — This relates to how long an athlete has been in a formal training program. Obviously, the athlete who has been in a formal training program for several years would be expected to have an advanced understanding of training elements and of the vocabulary of training compared to an athlete who has never been in such a program.

Competitive Schedule — Is it an extended or a concentrated competitive season?

Composition of the Team — Is it a team of more mature players with advanced training age or a team of novices?

Gender — The female athlete must devote a greater proportion of her training to strength training.

"24-Hour Athlete" Concept — The time away from training has a greater impact on performance and training than the relatively small amount of daily time devoted to training. Therefore, lifestyle, work, and school situations must be carefully considered.

Recovery — Carefully plan recovery between workouts and throughout the year-round plan to allow for adaptation.

The Block System

The solution to effectively planning and implementing year-round training is to take a "block approach." This allows you to identify specific objectives in order to address strengths and weaknesses in the individual player and the team. Each component of fitness must be included in each block. They are threaded throughout the training year based on the demands of the sport and the individual athlete's strengths and weaknesses as well as his or her stage of development. Blocks can be positioned in a training year as needed, or as demands dictate. Thus, once a block system has been put in place, such as a training plan that follows an individual past the regular competitive season and into a state tournament, it can be revised easily if the athlete or team does not make it past regionals.

The block system is a method of addressing the complex interaction between the development and stabilization of multiple physical capacities without compromising skill development, while providing time for adaptation. With the developing athlete, regardless of the block, growth and development must always be a prime consideration. Finally, when implementing such a system, it is important that the transition between blocks be seamless. One block must flow into the other without apparent, abrupt changes.

Testing and Evaluating — A key aspect of a good year-round training program is testing and evaluation. This is an ongoing process, not something that is done once or twice a year. Time and measure at every opportunity in order to ascertain progress. Remember that competition is the highest form of testing. At the developmental levels, however, if the game is the only measure of progress, there will never be enough games to show progress. ◆

Putting New Drills To the Test

There is no shortage of enticing new drills that you will learn about from clinics, conferences, and publications that you read. Many times, I have come back from training seminars with a new drill that seemed particularly useful until I put it into one of my training programs. More often than not, I found that the new drill did not do anything better than what I was doing, or in extreme cases, I found that the new drill was ineffective.

How do you know if a new drill or exercise is right for your program? The answer is that every drill you consider needs to be evaluated using several criteria. First, you need to evaluate the drill's effectiveness and determine its optimal placement within the context of your overall training program. Second, you need to analyze where the drill fits in your daily workouts.

Identify

Let's begin by looking at the first step, which is to identify the effective drills among all the new drills that you will come across. Begin by asking yourself some key questions about each new drill. These questions focus on WHAT the drill will accomplish, and WHY it would improve your program. Here is a checklist of questions you should ask about any drill under consideration:

- How is this drill performed? Review the mechanics of the new drill. You need to completely understand the drill to assess it. because correct execution will be essential for eliciting optimum training adaptation.
- What will this drill accomplish? Think of a drill as a precision instrument. It should have a specific application and training goal. Does this specific goal fit the needs of your program? If not, remove this drill from consideration.
- Why should I add this new drill to my program? Perhaps the most important question that a coach can ask is whether a drill is a "need to do" activity or a "nice to do" activity. If it is simply "nice," then it won't add anything to your program and it should not be included in your workouts. You should only add a drill if it fills a gap in your training or if it achieves an objective better than existing drills.
- What particular athletic component does the drill enhance? When you consider a drill, be very specific in identifying the exact athletic qualities or components that it will address. If it attempts to do too much, be wary of its effectiveness.
- Is the drill practical in your situation? For example, if you are training a 30-member team, specialized equipment needed for a drill may be too expensive to equip a whole team or it may take too much time to set up each day.
- What level of development is the drill suited for? Certain drills are better suited for developing athletes rather than more advanced athletes. Be sure to assess the drill with your particular athlete's developmental stage in mind.
- What are the ranges of sets and repetitions? Are the sets and repetitions congruent with the purpose of the drill? Do they achieve your goals for this drill?

Placing the Drill

If the new drill has survived to this point it is now time to think about placement of that drill. Putting a drill into a context that optimizes its effectiveness should be a key element in the design of any training program.

Proper placement means putting the drill into a daily workout so that it not only builds upon the drill that comes before it, but prepares the athlete for the drill that follows. Like an individual brick in a wall, a drill that is inserted in the proper time and place will strengthen and enhance the entire structure of the workout. If the drill does not fit anywhere in your program, then it is not appropriate for your needs. If it is placed improperly, it will be useless for your program.

Analyzing and placing a new drill is certainly not a black-and-white proposition. Each drill is unique, as is every coach's program. The key is understanding the variables that make up your program and thoroughly embracing the team goals.

Examples

Here are some new drills that I've fit into my training programs. I'll describe how I assessed them and decided they would be beneficial. I'll also explain how I placed them in the daily workout.

Stance Throw Drill — The starting stance for this drill can be a standing stance or a three- or four-point down stance. A medicine ball weighing three or four kilograms is placed on the ground directly in front of the athlete. Then, the athlete executes the drill by picking up the ball and simultaneously accelerating forward while throwing the ball outward. Measure the distance the ball is thrown and the time it takes the athlete to move a specific distance from the start, usually about ten yards.

I like this drill because it reinforces good starting mechanics and develops explosiveness while coming out of a down starting position that a football player would use. For football or rugby, this drill also enhances the ability to deliver a blow.

In order to obtain the full effect of this exercise, athletes should do this workout after they are warmed up, but are still fresh and have plenty of energy. Consequently, it should be placed in the beginning of a workout, after the warmup.

A new drill may seem great at a workshop, but how do you know if it will be good for your specific program?

Multi-Directional Jumps — The athlete begins by standing with the feet shoulder-width apart. He or she then executes a standing jump forward. Upon landing, the athlete immediately takes off again and jumps sideways, turning 90 degrees in the air. Then immediately take off again, jumping sideways and turning another 90 degrees in the air so that upon the next landing, the athlete faces the opposite direction of where he or she began. The athlete should then immediately take off and jump backward to finish.

Start by keeping the jumps short and gradually lengthening the distance jumped. Once the rhythm and technique of this sequence are mastered, have your athletes perform two consecutive series of the jump. Two series of jumps are considered one set. A typical multi-directional jumping drill will have the athlete execute three to five sets of jumps, depending on the overall objective of the workout.

This drill works great as a remedial plyometric exercise. It proprioceptively challenges the athlete and helps prevent knee injuries. This drill should be done early in the workout because its basic purpose is to warm up and strengthen the knees. Multi-directional jumps can be performed daily as long as the number of jumps is adjusted according to your athlete's abilities and your individual goals.

Standing Bench Press (stretch cord) — To begin, attach a stretch cord to each end of a wooden dowel, and securely attach the other ends of the cords to a pole or fence behind the athlete. The athlete grasps the dowel with two hands and positions the dowel at chest height so that all slack is taken out of the stretch cord. He or she begins the exercise in a good athletic stance with the feet shoulder-width apart and the knees slightly flexed. Then, the athlete presses the dowel outward as rapidly as possible using full range of motion. It is important to control the return (eccentric) phase to get the full benefit of this workout. Have the athlete perform three to five sets of 12 to 15 repetitions each.

While assessing this drill, I realized it was perfect for applying the strength developed in more traditional movements to a posture that is common to most sport situations. This exercise is also important because it enables you to integrate strength training and core stability in a way that will not occur if you are doing presses while lying on a weight bench or strapped into a machine.

The standing bench press is considered a transitional upper-body strength exercise, so I usually couple it with a variety of bench presses and medicine ball chest passes. It is a companion to upper-body strength drills such as push-ups and regular bench presses and should be placed in a sequence with them.

One of the reasons everyone likes new drills is that they are fun. Giving your athletes something different and unique makes the workout more motivational, which often leads to better effort and better results.

BOSU™ Squat Sequence — A BOSU™ can be described as half a stability ball attached to a plastic base. The BOSU™ is one of several new training devices designed to challenge balance and proprioception in an environment of controlled instability.

I chose BOSU™ exercises because I was looking for something that prepares the nervous system for more complex activities. It should be placed early in a daily workout, preferably leading into resistance squats. There are many drills that can be centered on the BOSU™ device, but the three that I frequently use are included below in a sequence of squats. These drills are effective for sports such as basketball or soccer, where an athlete has to perform reciprocal leg actions.

Squat on one BOSU™ — Have the athlete stand on the BOSU™ with a relatively narrow stance with his or her hands placed on the hips, so that the arms cannot be used for counter balance. He or she should perform a normal squat, completing two sets of 20 repetitions.

Squat on two BOSU™ — The BOSU™ are placed next to each other, and the athlete places one foot on top of each BOSU™. Have the athlete perform two sets of 20 repetitions.

Squat down on two BOSU™ and up on one BOSU™ — Again use the two BOSU™, but in this exercise have the athlete shift to just one leg on the ascent. He or she should alternate legs for each repetition. Have the athlete perform two sets of 20 reps.

Increasing Demand Runs — The idea behind this drill is to progressively increase the effort of the run from a comfortable aerobic pace up to a mixed aerobic/anaerobic effort that approaches 90 percent effort. Along with developing aerobic power, the objective of this drill is to teach athletes to monitor their bodies and to control their runs by controlling their efforts.

I have found this drill especially useful for the non-endurance athlete and the team sport athlete who does not know how to distribute running effort to get a good aerobic training effect. It is a good "meat and potato" drill that can be the focus of a daily workout. It should be placed in the middle of a workout, after an athlete is totally warmed up but still has plenty of energy.

Give careful consideration to the time increments, as well as the total duration of the run. Usually, two sets of nine to 12 minutes are very effective. This is a relatively sophisticated drill that may not be appropriate for novice athletes.

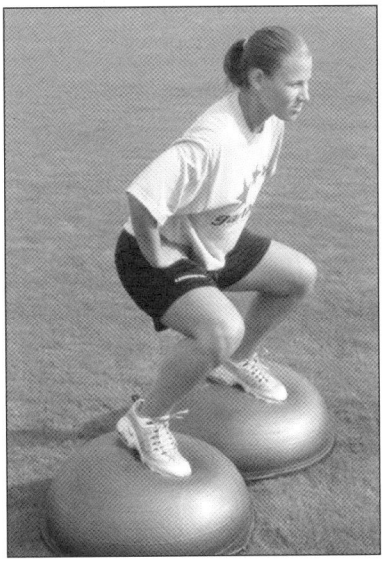
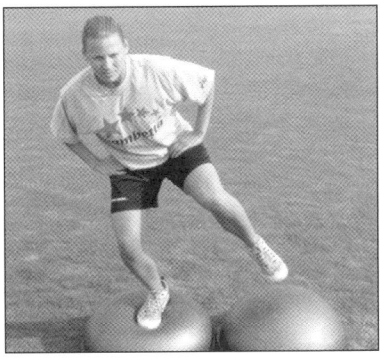
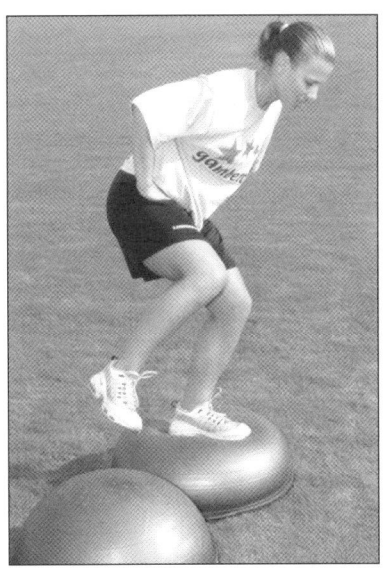

Drills on the BOSU™ can challenge an athlete's balance and proprioception in an environment of controlled instability. In this sequence, an athlete squats on two BOSU™ then shifts to one leg on the ascent.

Progressions

One of the reasons everyone likes new drills is that they are fun. Giving your athletes something different and unique makes the workout more motivational, which often leads to better effort and better results. But finding a new drill to replace something already existing in your program is not so easy.

A better way to keep things fresh is to progress some of your tried-and-true drills in interesting ways. For example, if one wants to build an athlete's lower extremity with a basic squat exercise, a progression of drills can be instituted as the athlete's legs and lower back become stronger. There really is limit to where you can go with this progression. It is dictated to you by the demands of the sport, by the athlete's position within the sport, and by the qualities of the individual athlete.

Below, I provide an example of a progression with a squat that would take three to four weeks to complete and leads the squat toward the direction of a total-body exercise. It begins with the body weight squat and progresses to squats with external resistance as the athlete's strength increases. Once each variation of the squat is learned, that variation is plugged into later workouts as needed. This particular progression is useful for training during the off-season because it begins with a modest challenge and builds from there. Try to begin with 20 repetitions in the following drills, but remember, as external resistance increases, repetitions and speed should decrease.

Body Weight Squat — Hands interlocked behind the head. Execute a full squat at one rep per second.

Weight Vest Squat — The body perceives this drill as an internal load. Otherwise, the emphasis is the same as the previous squat.

Sand Bag Squat — A tubular sandbag is draped over the athlete's shoulders. This added resistance will slow movement down, but the sandbag will still be perceived by the body as an internal load.

Dumbbell Squat — Have the athlete squat while holding a dumbbell at each shoulder.

Dumbbell Squat To Press — Have the athlete squat down and press the dumbbells up on the ascent.

Dumbbell Shift Squat — Have the athlete squat down on two legs and then shift to one leg for the ascent. He or she should alternate legs.

Dumbbell Shift Squat To Press — Have the athlete squat down on two legs, then shift to one leg for the ascent and perform a press with the opposite arm.

Note that I do not recommend how much weight is used with each example above. That factor depends on the athlete and the sport being played. For example, a soccer player would not have to overcome the external resistance that a football player normally does. As a result, football players would train with more external resistance than most soccer players.

There is no shortage of drills available to you. Remember, the key is using each drill for a specific purpose within the context of the whole training program. Try to make drills fit into a workout so that there is a logical flow from one to another. This process demands a clear understanding of the objectives of the entire training program as well as the application of each drill. Remember, a program with a few well thought-out, well-placed drills is far better than a program that is haphazardly packed with drills just to fill time. ◆

The Daily Special

Attention to detail is a concept that is synonymous with success. In the conditioning world, attention to detail means emphasizing the most basic element in any successful training plan: the individual training session. A long-term training plan is essentially a succession of individual training sessions linked in pursuit of specific objectives. And because each session is an integral building block for the whole training program, it should receive the greatest amount of attention in planning. In other words, planning the details of individual sessions will determine the success of your long-term training goals.

The first detail that you need to plan is the theme of each session. A training session must have a general theme, such as an emphasis on speed and acceleration, lateral speed and agility, conditioning, strength, or endurance. This theme creates a cohesiveness between the drills within that daily session. For example, if you are emphasizing speed, you need to choose drills that build speed and naturally flow into one another. In addition, the task of creating a theme for each training session forces you to consider what components are necessary to reach your long-term training goals.

Each theme, in turn, should have very specific and measurable objectives. For example, objectives of speed and acceleration are easily measured and recorded using a stopwatch, while strength can be quantified by recording the amount of external resistance and repetitions. You must be able to measure and record progress in order to determine whether your overall objectives are being met.

Teach, Train, or Maintain

Once you choose a general theme for each training session, you need to group sessions into three areas of emphasis: sessions with a teaching emphasis, sets of sessions with a training emphasis, and sessions with a maintenance emphasis.

Sessions with a teaching or a training emphasis will require significantly more time than maintenance workouts, particularly early in the season when building athletes' skills and conditioning levels is the major concern.

Workouts with a teaching emphasis are primarily designed to build an athlete's understanding of skills and therefore, they are more time consuming. If an athlete doesn't "get it," be patient, spend the extra time, and be sure that he or she does eventually learn the skill, drill, or exercise.

When training a group, carefully plan to meet individual needs in a group context. Everyone will not progress and learn at the same rate. Remember not to rush your athletes through these sessions. Instead, take time to attend to the smallest details of the session.

Attention to detail in daily training sessions spells success for your long-term conditioning program.

Workouts with a training emphasis should be part of a refining process that is designed to improve the basic skills that were taught in the teaching emphasis workouts. Remember, refining skills already taught will involve more repetition (the old adage, "practice makes permanent" comes into play here).

Once the season begins, or once your athletes' conditioning and skills reach desired levels, the emphasis should change from sessions that focus on teaching and refining to those that emphasize the maintenance, or stabilization, of what your athletes have already learned. The idea here is to maintain specific playing skills along with the levels of strength and conditioning that have been attained thus far.

Conducting maintenance workouts once the competitive season begins is practical for several reasons. First, you want to avoid the possibility of causing overuse injuries and wearing down athletes who are facing the rigors of regular competition. Therefore, maintenance workouts should be intense with significantly less volume and duration than the early-season workouts that emphasized the development of strength, speed, and skills. Moreover, once a season begins, the time has passed for teaching basic skills. Your in-season emphasis should instead be keeping your athletes in shape, focused, and motivated.

Long-Range Focus

While you are planning the details of individual sessions and even individual drills, never forget that every component of each session must pursue the specific objectives of the workout. Always remember that the session is not an end in itself, but a means to an end.

I have found that using a modular training concept helps maintain a focus on the long-term plan when working on the details of the short-term, individual session. The training module concept is quite simple: design combinations and sequences of compatible exercises all geared to the theme of each session. In other words, an individual teaching session with an emphasis on endurance should entail a module of aerobic-emphasis exercises. Similarly, a session that focuses on building explosive strength should contain modules of interrelated drills that include external resistance and plyometrics.

Within each module, exercises should be carefully sequenced to flow from one to the next. The volume and intensity for the exercises within each module are based on an analysis of the previous session. This analysis should include the conditioning levels of your athletes, how effective the drills are, and whether the particular module is implemented preseason or in-season. Also, whether you are creating workouts for in-season or

Strength Theme

These are examples of two sessions with an overall theme of increasing a basketball player's basic strength. The emphasis is to develop the athlete's ability to handle his or her own bodyweight, then to be able to handle an external resistance of dumbbells and free weights. In terms of power, the focus is on teaching and stabilization of jumping techniques, especially landing techniques as a precursor to an emphasis on lateral speed and agility in the pre-season training phase.

Each workout begins with a warm-up that emphasizes fundamental movements (coordination and balance) and core strength. There is no conditioning work during this phase, although the athletes should be playing summer league games and having informal practices. Strength and power development along with individual skill development is the player's focus.

Monday

Group One: Mini band routine
    Basic Core Drills:
        1) Wide 2) Tight 3) Over the top 4) Figure eight

    Multi-Dimensional Stretch:
        1) Lunge reach series 2) Jack knife crawl
        3) Creepy crawl 4) Hurdle walks

    Coordination:
        1) Skip 2) Side step 3) Carioca
        4) Backward run 5) High skip

    Balance (hold each position 10 seconds):
        1) Single-leg squat balance 2) Balance shift
        3) Balance circuit

    Strength Training:
        Incline push-up 4 x 10
        Incline pull-up 4 x 12 (feet elevated)
        Combo I (curl and press) 3 x 6
        Combo II (over the top) 2 x 6
        Standing bench press 3 x 12
        Bent row 4 x 6
        Reverse fly 3 x 12
        Arm step-ups 3 x 20

    Medicine Ball Wall Throws:
        Overhead throw 20 x
        Soccer throw 20 x
        Chest pass 20 x
        Down the side 20 x
        Cross in front 20 x
        Around the back 20 x

Monday

Group Two: Mini band routine
    Basic Core Drills:
        1) Wide 2) Tight 3) Over the top 4) Figure eight

    Multi-Dimensional Stretch:
        1) Reach series 2) Jack knife
        3) Creepy crawl 4) Hurdle walks

    Coordination:
        1) Skip 2) Side step 3) Carioca
        4) Backward run 5) High skip

    Balance (hold each position 10 seconds):
        1) Single-leg squat balance 2) Balance shift
        3) Balance circuit

    Plyometrics:
        Multi-direction jump 4x
        Lateral bound 3 x 10
        Hurdle jumps a) forward. 5x5
        b) Multi-directional 3x5
        Box-up jumps Forward, lateral and
        rotational 1 x 5 for each jump

    Strength Training:
        High pull 4 x 6
        Push jerk 4 x 6
        Leg circuit, three complete circuits (no recovery)
        Squat 20 x
        Lunge 20 x
        Step-up 20 x
        Jump squat 10 x

    Medicine Ball. Total Body Throws:
        Over-the-back throw 6 x
        Single-leg squat throw 6 x
        Forward through-the-leg 6 x
        Single squat scoop throw 6 x
        Squat throw 10 x

off-season use, make sure to include an injury prevention component. This component is most easily addressed in the warm-up through specific exercises and by integrating recovery times between individual sessions and drills. Consider how to incorporate recovery given the constraints of most situations. Self-massage, shaking, and stretching as well as intra-workout nutrition in the form of hydration are the most basic and practical forms of intra workout recovery.

Change of Season

Although conditioning coaches constantly change sessions to fit evolving program goals, I find it useful to use basic, proven templates for sessions. With a little tinkering, these templates can be used both in-season and off-season. My basic templates are listed below:

In-Season Template:

For an in-season daily plan, include the following elements:
- Warm-up. For an in-season workout, I focus my warm-up exercises on coordination, balance, and flexibility.
- Athletic Development Activity. This is the meat-and-potatoes of your workout. It includes all drills and exercises that you want your athletes to perform, minus the warm-up and cool-down. I divide my drills and exercises here into the following focuses: skill, tactics, strategy, and specific fitness drills such as leg strength or arm conditioning.
- Cooldown.

The following three templates are useful for off-season sessions. Within each template, arrange the drill sequences in the order listed:

Off-Season Template A: speed and acceleration theme.
- Warm-up with emphasis on coordination, balance, and flexibility
- Speed and Acceleration Work
- Lateral Speed and Agility Footwork
- Plyometrics
- Sport-specific Skill Work
- Strength Training
- Cooldown

Off-Season Template B: Lateral speed and agility theme.
- Warm-up
- Speed and Acceleration Work
- Lateral Speed and Agility Work
- Skill Work with the Ball
- Strength Training
- Cooldown

Off-Season Template C: Conditioning Theme.
- Continuous Warm-up
- Skill Work with the Ball
- Conditioning — Include intensive tempo, extensive tempo, or speed endurance
- Cooldown

Management Considerations

The details included in planning individual workouts go well beyond a list of exercises that athletes will follow. Other factors that have to be considered include training time available, size of the facility relative to the number of athletes, available equipment, available coaching personnel, and the number of athletes who will participate in the actual training session.

The following example of a training program for a female high school basketball team illustrates some of these management considerations. Because of the size and experience of the team, the athletes were divided into two groups, which allowed workouts to be staggered to accommodate limited practice space. This division also allowed more than one session for each group in a single day. Splitting a team may not be an ideal arrangement in terms of sequence of training, but in this case, it was expedient, practical, and it produced results.

In situations where multiple sessions in a day are used, it is helpful to use the following model of the focused workout for each session:

Focused Training Session: Everything is subservient to the focus of the workout. In this example the focus is on speed development.
- Warm-up
- Power Development: multi-jumps or multi-throws
- Speed Development
- Cooldown

A more typical scenario is using a complex training session once a day. It is called complex because it addresses multiple components within a single training session. It is common in team sports.

Complex Training Session:
- Warm-up
- Technical and Tactical Work
- Conditioning and Metabolic Work
- Strength Training
- Cooldown

Finally, at the conclusion of each session, the day's activities must be carefully evaluated and, if necessary, the sessions that follow it must be adjusted accordingly. Evaluation is a constant, ongoing process that should be part of each training session. Never lose sight of the fact that the ultimate test is the competition itself. ◆

Other factors that should be considered include training time, facility size, equipment, coaching personnel, and the number of athletes.

Team Training

It may be a cliche, but it doesn't make it any less true: A team is like a chain—it is only as strong as its weakest link. When it comes to conditioning a team, therefore, you must work toward making every single link as strong as possible.

But how can one devise a successful conditioning plan that will work in a large group setting? How do you raise the fitness level of the most fit while not overtraining the least fit? How do you take into account the pitcher's need for more shoulder exercises while also acknowledging the outfielder's need for more speed work?

First of all, don't disregard the essential conditioning theories of periodization, proper work-rest ratios, and testing and evaluation. All the tried-and-true theories that work in a one-on-one or small group setting must still be your guide.

The next step is adapting these conditioning principles in a large, often disparate, group. If your resources were endless, every athlete in the group would be treated individually—with an individualized plan and specific coach by his or her side. This, of course, is impossible in a high school or college setting. On the other side of the spectrum, it is tempting to have every team member follow the exact same workout regimen. This scenario, however, means you'd be affecting only a minority of the athletes, bringing the well-conditioned athletes down a notch and possibly injuring the out-of-shape athletes. The strategy that I've found works best is a happy medium between these two extremes. I break the team into smaller groups, based on their needs, then devise specific plans for each group. This allows athletes to have workouts tailored to their needs, but does not take too much extra time and resources. It is especially effective during the preseason and in-season periods, when time is at a premium and conditioning tends to get neglected unless it is included as part of the actual practice.

Analyze the Sport
Just as you would do when conditioning an individual athlete, the initial stage of your team plan is to analyze the demands of the sport. Most team sports can be divided into two broad categories: intermittent sprint sports and transition game sports.

Intermittent sprint sports, like football or baseball, are characterized by intense bouts of work, usually in very short bursts of three to five seconds in duration, followed by rest periods at least three to five times as long. Transition game sports, like soccer or lacrosse, are characterized by virtually continuous action in which there are brief periods of higher-intensity activity. There are very few breaks in the action, just changes in intensity of effort. Of course, not all sports follow those two models exactly. Basketball is one exception, as the action stops for time-outs or free-throw situations. Nonetheless, it has more of the characteristics of a transition game sport than an intermittent sprint sport.

Once we thoroughly evaluate and understand the sport's requirements, we must then take the next step, which is to understand the demands of the various positions within the sport. Each has different demands in terms of movement patterns, speed, strength, stamina, and so forth. Admittedly, this makes the training process more complicated, but it is critical to obtaining on-the-field results.

When it comes to conditioning a team, the best approach is to consider it as a collection of individuals.

In fact, the biggest mistake that we make is to condition all positions the same. A quarterback in football should not have the same strength-training program and tests as an offensive or defensive lineman. A forward in soccer has significantly different demands than a defensive midfielder. Therefore, we must look carefully at both the overall game and the requirements of the multiplicity of positions, and condition accordingly.

Evaluate and Group
Before doing any specific planning, it is also critical to understand the qualities each individual athlete brings to the respective sport and his or her individual position. Although it does take some time, evaluating each player is a must. Test each athlete on his or her endurance, speed, and all qualities specific to the sport and his or her position.

These evaluations then allow you to properly group each athlete into training teams. The key to making these groups work is to keep them dynamic. By that, I mean that the composition of the group is dependent upon the physical quality you are training. For example, an athlete could be in one group for speed-development work and an entirely different group for strength training. In addition, an athlete could switch groups if he or she is advancing more quickly than others in the group.

At first glance, it may seem that this approach would make conditioning a team more complicated. But in fact, it makes it much easier to define programs and assign individuals to groups to accomplish specific tasks. It takes a little more work up front, but it really makes the process much more manageable.

A Yearly Plan
How do you structure the training year for a team? The key is to look at the in-season competitive schedule, then build everything to point toward this. Make note

of the dates of key competitions, then work backwards. Look at the time available before those competitions and break that time into manageable blocks with themes or objectives for each block.

Your major focus should be on the off-season and pre-season training times, which is when you'll want to steadily increase workloads. In season it is preferable to under-train and keep athletes more fresh. However, at all times, there should be a real emphasis on monitoring the effects of training in order to get an optimal return.

Therefore, it is very important to develop a good system for accountability. Measure, time, and record every workout possible. Make sure that the athletes get feedback on their results and that the coaching staff and trainers are also kept apprised of training results. Document everything! Keep detailed records of each athlete's attendance at conditioning workouts as well as compliance and effort during the workouts.

Working with Other Staff

A key to effective work in conditioning a team is communication. I know this is another overused term, but it is essential. There must be clear, open lines of communication with the head coach, coaching staff, athletic trainer, and the medical staff as to the health status of the players. This is true of equipment people as well, particularly if there are any special equipment needs. And don't forget the groundskeepers, as they can make your job a whole lot easier. Of course, it is the coaching staff whom you'll need to communicate with most often. It is essential that you talk to them about how much of the work the players will be doing with the sport coaches might overlap with what you are planning to do with conditioning. The best idea is to always be at practice so that you can gauge the intensity of the practice. What the players are doing at sport practice may cause you to adjust the volume or intensity of the work you have planned for post-practice or even for the next day.

Conditioning coaches know that for most of the year, the team is not under their control. The focus of training in most phases is on the technical, tactical, and strategic considerations. Conditioning must fit around those aspects. That may not be the ideal, but it is the reality. In other words, in addition to communicating with the coaches, make sure your conditioning plans are somewhat flexible. For effective athletic conditioning, it is vital to have a good sound plan. But, when it comes to working with a team sport, it is also important to have a detailed contingency plan.

Athletes Come First

Above all, we must be able to communicate effectively with the athletes. Identify key athletes who will give you honest feedback about the training. Understand who will cry wolf at the easiest workout or who is the workhorse who can never get enough. Seek out feedback from all types of players in order to make the conditioning more effective. It's also important to let them discover their athleticism. Although teaching correct mechanics is important, be careful not to over-coach and make them robots. Allow them to discover patterns of movement that work for them. Encourage creativity though pressure situations where the player has to make fast decisions at "game speed." In addition, let the members of each training group push one another and work together. Try to keep the play element in conditioning without making it frivolous. One workout cannot make an athlete, but one workout can break an athlete. What that tells us is, with a team, we must always keep the big picture in mind. Each element of a practice is more than an exercise or a workout. We must understand where it fits into the context of the team's long-term conditioning development. ◆

Providing Structure

The following structure is particularly effective in team-sport settings.
1. The whole team does a general warm-up together. This should take about 10-15 minutes.
2. Athletes break into groups, emphasizing very specific components of training. Each group goes through two stations a day with 8 - 10 minutes assigned to each station.

The stations are as follows:
A. Straight-ahead speed: acceleration work
B. Lateral speed and agility
C. Specific speed: actual movements of the game
D. Core work
E. Plyometrics
F. Balance

Each station has a set number of drills in a prescribed progression. The emphasis is always on quality of movement and effort. Each drill has a prescribed number of sets and reps. In this context, it is also possible to work on individual weaknesses by repeating a station for emphasis. It is best to set up the rotation so that the athletes do two stations per day. Therefore, the pattern for the training for one group for a week without a game would look like this:

Day #1	Day #2	Day #3	Day #4	Day #5	Day #6
A/B	C/D	E/F	A/B	C/D	E/F

Breaking Through Plateaus

How often has it happened that you'll be training a group of athletes and one or more of them will hit a plateau in their performance? Their efforts in both workouts and competitions aren't getting any worse, but no matter how hard they train, they're just not improving.

Usually, the athlete's reaction is one of panic. "What's going on? What will I do now?" But, rather than being cause for concern, on the contrary, it's important to realize that once an athlete has been training for any period of time, it is inevitable that he or she will hit a performance plateau. In fact, if you haven't witnessed this phenomenon, there may be something wrong with your training program.

What exactly is a plateau? It is a temporary stagnation or slight decline in performance or training. It is important to point out that a plateau in performance is not the same as overtraining. Overtraining is a very negative outcome of many factors, which ultimately results in a significant decline in performance and/or the capacity to train. It involves extreme fatigue, failure in training and competition, and psychologically, the athlete does not want to train or compete.

Plateaus, on the other hand, are a normal part of training progression. Performance improvement and training progress are not linear. There will be periods of stagnation, just as there will be periods of rapid improvement. (Hopefully, there will not be periods of regression, but sometimes that is also the case.)

Ideally, in any training year and throughout an athletic lifetime, performance improves as a staircase-like series of ever-ascending small plateaus leading to a period of peak performance. Each step in the staircase is a period of adaptation to the stimulus of the previous training period. If we can evaluate our progress in this light, and we can control the duration of each plateau, then the plateau can be seen as it should be viewed: as a very positive training phenomenon.

By controlling the training process, the lifestyle, and the competition schedule, it is possible to control the plateaus. This requires careful planning and monitoring of day-to-day training as well as execution of a good long-term plan. The athlete must be fully aware of his or her role in the whole process, and provide objective, ongoing feedback to help the coach make any necessary adjustments.

What are the causes of plateaus? Generally, plateaus result from too much time spent in a particular mode, routine, or training environment. For example, carrying out a heavy lifting cycle for six weeks with the same sets and reps done on the same training days will certainly lead to a plateau. Athletes in sports with extended competitive seasons, like baseball, basketball, and tennis, are particularly susceptible to extended plateaus.

The competition schedule can play a significant role in the cause of plateaus. Too little or too much competition can cause a plateau in performance. The former can make the athlete feel like the training lacks a purpose, while the latter does not give the athlete enough time to train and prepare. Also, competition against an inferior opponent will often result in a stagnation of performance, because the athlete is not challenged, and neither the training nor the competition offer enough stimulus for adaptation to occur.

Remember that training is a cumulative process. No one workout or training method will make all the difference—the total of all the components is what determines the ultimate training adaptation. That is why it

> ... Start with seeing plateaus for what they are – natural periods in the training progression – and institute change before athletes get stuck in a rut.

Table One: Variety Is the Spice of Life

Varying the patterns of work from week to week can keep athletes from getting stuck in plateaus as well as help them break out of plateaus.

Week One

Monday		Wednesday		Friday
speed & power		power & speed		strength & fitness

Week Two

Monday	Tuesday		Thursday	Friday
Speed	Power		strength	fitness

Week Three

Monday	Tuesday		Thursday	Friday
speed	power		fitness	strength

is so important to plan and recognize the plateau phenomenon for what it is—just a part of the normal process of adaptation. Too often, we take a microscopic approach, which blows one exercise, training session, or game out of proportion to the whole training program. A macro approach will go a long way to putting each session in the context of the whole plan.

So, how can you help your athletes break through plateaus and move on to the next level of performance? The simplest solution is to carefully plan their training and competition. Be sure to build into the training plan frequent changes in the training stimulus, the training routine, and the training environment. In the plan, pay particular attention to the sequence of work so that training components are complementary. Carefully control the volume and intensity of the total workload as well as the individual components of training. Plan competitions so that there is a good mix in terms of degree of difficulty, as well as adequate time between competitions to allow for full recovery and training. (Although coaches generally do not have much control over their regular-season in-league schedules, they do have a fair amount of control over their non-league schedules, exhibition games, scrimmages, etc.)

There are many ways to change a training program to avoid prolonged plateaus or to break a plateau. The key is that each of the changes must have a specific purpose and methodology. When looking at changes in the training program, it is helpful to break them up as either little changes or big changes.

The Big Changes

Volume — The total training load. Volume can either be increased or decreased. It is generally agreed that no more than a ten percent increase or reduction in work is recommended from any one training period to the next.

Speed — The rate at which the individual exercises or the training regimen are performed can be varied.

Rest interval — Rest as a variable needs to be considered both intra-workout and inter-workout. Intra-workout refers to decreasing or increasing the rest between exercises or drills, which can significantly change the training demand and emphasis. Inter-workout rest can include strategies such as adding another recovery or an active rest day to the weekly training cycle. Remember that it is during rest that adaptation occurs.

Training mode — This can be changed by using a little creativity. For example, in squats you can use body weight, a weight vest, a bar, dumbbells, do squat jumps, back squats, front squats, or overhead squats. The movements and muscles are all similar, but the stimulus is varied enough that the body will perceive each exercise as different. This will prevent an athlete from getting stuck in a plateau and help him or her to break out of a plateau.

Training sequences — Modify the sequence of training to achieve optimum results. For example, within a workout, place your plyometric work after weights or have your athletes weight train and then do sprints. Also, look carefully at your sequence during the training week. It is important to have several different patterns of work, so that you can change the order of the primary stimulus focus for the days of the week. This change of sequence can have a very significant effect on the control of the plateau.

Environment — Move from outdoors to indoors or vice versa, or change the training surface.

The Little Changes

Balance — Challenge the proprioceptive system. Have your athletes close their eyes, perform exercises on a soft surface, or train barefoot.

Visual feedback — Altering the visual feedback — anything from the color of the walls or the carpet to the placement of the championship flags or posters on the walls — changes the stimulus and helps break the routine.

Kinesthetic awareness — Go from a thin bar to a fat bar or a padded bar. Go from a medicine ball to a powerball.

Cues — Change cues from verbal to visual or kinesthetic, or vary the cues within a given training session.

Nature of the drill (closed or open response) — A closed drill has only one predetermined response and

Table Two: Remedy for Every Plateau

Types of Plateaus	Remedies
Speed (speed barrier)	Assisted speed drills Resisted speed drills More quality, less volume More rest Better hydration ($1/3$-1 oz per pound of body weight per day)
Strength	Less volume (fewer sets, fewer reps) More load Same volume (more sets, fewer reps)
Size	Greater or same load More volume Less volume Better nutrition More rest
Work Capacity	More volume Less rest Better nutrition Better hydration

the athlete can focus on the required motor skill or technique. With an open drill, there are a variety of possible responses.

In general, it is possible to improve the quality of work by increasing the rest, changing the load, varying the tempo of the exercise, altering the intensity, changing the speed, raising or lowering the arousal level, or narrowing or broadening the focus. For every type of plateau, altering one or more of these factors will help your athletes get through it.

The main thing is to recognize plateaus for what they are: normal adaptive responses to training. When your athletes hit a plateau, it is important to reassure them of this and help guide them safely out. You can use any of the above-mentioned methods to help your athletes avoid prolonged plateaus or to break through them. Having a good plan will go a long way toward controlling the plateau phenomenon. ◆

The Perils Of Overtraining

In order to excel, athletes must push themselves. Sometimes, it is even necessary to push to the edge. But, where exactly is the edge? And how can athletes know when they are pushing themselves too far or too hard? When an athlete pushes too hard for too long, not only will performance stop improving, it will very quickly start to deteriorate. Once an athlete has gone from training to overtraining, it's not just performance that falters — his or her health suffers as well. Then it's a long, hard road back. In most cases, the athlete's competitive season is lost. If a problem is not spotted quickly enough, the athlete can be at serious risk for significant emotional and physical damage. Thus, it is crucial that every athlete, coach, and athletic trainer be able to identify this overtrained state and the markers leading to it.

In many respects, however, this area of training is unexplored territory. Even as we better understand the body and its adaptive mechanisms, there remains much confusion regarding the signs of overtraining and what to do to reverse the effects. What most professionals in the field do agree on is that the best remedy for overtraining is prevention, and fortunately there is a fair amount of consensus on how this can be done.

What Is Overtraining?

One of the biggest problems is defining exactly what overtraining is. It has also been referred to as burnout, and conditions such as chronic fatigue syndrome may be related to overtraining. One thing we know for sure is that overtraining is more than normal fatigue or feeling tired. It first manifests as trouble with technique and performance errors and is followed by performance decline. Sometimes, the initial stage is so subtle as to be virtually unnoticeable. The next stage is a gradual onset of persistent joint and muscle soreness. Conditions such as swimmer's shoulder, jumper's knee, or Achilles tendinitis become nagging problems.

In the early stages of overtraining, there will also be a decrease in appetite, with an accompanying loss of body weight. In most cases, the overtrained athlete will be more susceptible to colds, fevers, sore throats, and possibly allergic reactions. Also, tenderness, soreness, and swelling of the lymph nodes often occurs. Lethargy away from workouts is quite common, as are excessive and profuse sweating with minimal exertion, and shortness of breath during the warm-up or the feeling that the warm-up takes as much effort as a workout. Irritability toward people and situations that do not normally cause agitation is another sign. Table One lists the major markers of overtraining.

Overtraining is caused by a series of problems—a chain reaction of scenarios that, if not stopped early enough, can easily spiral out of control. While not caused by one milestone event, overtraining is characterized by a drastic, unexpected decline in the athlete's capacity to train and compete.

Overtraining is different from plateauing, which is recognized as a normal part of the training process. It should also not be confused with "over-reaching,"—is a term that has come into use the past ten years to describe a slight decline in performance due to the normal stress of training. Overreaching is a normal part of the adaptive process. In fact, if adequate recovery is timed properly as part of a plan, over-reaching is followed by a super-compensation effect, which is a positive adaptation. In my opinion, over-reaching is a term that has no place in the lexicon of training.

One workout cannot make an athlete, but one workout can break an athlete.

Essentially, overtraining results from a failure to consider the processes of training and recovery as an inseparable, unified whole. As such, it is also important to consider the athlete's life outside of his or her training — those 20 to 22 hours each day may be more important than what they do when training.

The developing athlete who is trying to balance school, relationships, work, family responsibilities, and training is very susceptible to overtraining. In looking back on athletes I have coached who were overtrained, it is clear that aspects of their lives outside of training probably were major contributing factors. It was a failure on my part to recognize these factors and adjust training and competition accordingly that further contributed to the overtrained state. Table Two lists some of the common causes of overtraining.

Very often, overtraining is closely related to self-image and self-concept — a prime candidate is the insecure athlete with a poor self-image who wants to do that little extra and pushes him- or herself over the edge. The things that make an athlete successful are the same things that lead to overtraining — an insatiable desire to succeed. But, it is more than a willingness to work, it is actually an obsession with work. The most at-risk athletes tend to be wrestlers and distance runners. Women are at a higher risk than men. Not surprisingly, these are the same populations who are most at-risk for eating disorders.

Is overtraining different for the speed/power athlete than the endurance athlete? Generally, the endurance athlete is more susceptible to overtraining than the speed and power athlete, simply because of the emphasis on volume in the endurance athlete's training. That is not to imply that the speed/power athlete does not get overtrained. More often than not, the speed/power athlete's overtraining is the result of too great a volume of high-intensity work. When the speed/power athlete reaches an overtrained state, the effect is even more dramatic, because of

Table One: What are the markers of overtraining?

Quality of sleep: Restless, interrupted sleep is a good indicator. Another sign is if the athlete wakes up tired.

Training attitude: If the athlete does not look forward to training.

Appetite: Generally, a loss of appetite is a sign. I have also found abnormal cravings for certain foods to be a sign.

Bodyweight: Has the athlete had unusual gains or losses, or wide fluctuations in weight?

Joint and muscle soreness: Muscle soreness that declines after a day or two is normal. Persistent soreness is not normal. Joint soreness, especially if it persists, is not good.

Training performances: Inability to complete workouts that formerly were done with ease.

Competition results: If there is a large drop-off in performance over several competitions, this is usually a powerful indicator.

Less-Reliable Markers

Pulse-rate: This is not as reliable a marker of overtraining as once thought. There are too many variables that can affect heart rate, even a.m. resting heart rate. Intra-workout heart rate can be useful to monitor recovery between workouts. This can be a good yardstick in sports with a high cardiovascular demand, but is not particularly valuable for the speed/power athlete.

Blood measures: This invasive measure is expensive and not readily available to most coaches and athletes. Further, no consistent blood markers have been found to be good predictors.

Urinalysis: This also is not readily available in most situations. Therefore, it is not practical.

---

the explosive nature of the events. The events are usually measured in very small increments; therefore, any overtraining will be dramatically magnified.

Also, it is less likely that a team-sport athlete will be overtrained when he or she is training with the team. It seems that if there is a positive group energy and environment, then overtraining is less likely to occur. I have seen several overtrained teams but most of it was related to a coach who did not understand the need for recovery and variability in training.

Prevention Is the Best Medicine

Current literature and my own experience substantiate that the best prescription for overtraining is prevention. Careful consideration needs to be given to training loads, recovery time, training modalities, and most importantly, the competitive schedule. The old adage that an ounce of prevention is worth a pound of cure could not be more true.

First and foremost, we must get past our incessant obsession with training volumes. More is not better. In many sports, especially the speed and power sports, volume is not the stimulus for specific adaptation, intensity is. In the same vein, it is imperative to remember that training is cumulative. No one session or week of training will make an athlete's career, but it can break it.

Training expert Thomas Kurz, in his excellent book, *Science and Sport of Training*, states that overtraining has more to do with the sequence of work than the total training load. Improper sequence leads to excessive overload by not allowing the body to adequately recover. The best way to prevent overtraining, therefore, is to have a good plan. The following provides a good foundation:

- Never increase volume and intensity at the same time.
- Always allow adequate recovery time — both intra-workout (between bouts of exercise) and inter-workout (between workout sessions).
- Make sure that the diet is well-balanced and appropriate to the training and sport demands.
- Adapt the training to the environmental conditions.
- Where possible, control life-stress demands.
- Individualize the training — no two individuals will respond to the stress of training the same way.
- Closely monitor competitive stress.

It is impossible to improve as an athlete without a certain threshold of training stress. As the athlete begins to train harder (especially the younger, developing athlete), the improvement is usually commensurate with the increase in training. But eventually, there is a point of diminishing returns, where increasing the workload will not necessarily lead to further improvement. It is at this juncture that the components of the program must be balanced and rest and recovery must be carefully planned in order for the athlete to realize continued improvement. Generally, this will occur between the training ages of four and six years. (Training age, as opposed to chronological age, refers to the amount of time an athlete has been in a formal, systematic training program.)

At this stage, and thereafter, it is important to continue to carefully balance all the various elements of training. According to Brent Rushall, a professor of sports psychology at San Diego State University and renowned expert in conditioning, as well as other experts, one of the best ways to monitor and measure an athlete's status when he or she may be on the brink of overtraining is to simply ask him or her for a subjective rating of how he or she feels. This, coupled with close observations by the coaches, will go a long way toward preventing overtraining. Remember that by the time the physiological indicators show up, the level of training is probably already approaching overtraining. Rushall also feels that the psychological factors better predict the onset of overtraining than do the physiological factors, because psychological disturbances occur prior to measurable physiological indicators.

It is very important for all athletes—not just those on the

brink of overtraining—and their coaches to closely monitor athletes' training and their responses to the training. There are subjective measures—in essence, a scan of the body—that each individual athlete has to monitor daily. Coaches should require each of their athletes to keep a detailed training diary for the athlete's own personal use. I have also found it useful, especially with student-athletes, to give them a seven-day monitoring sheet that asks them to report hours of sleep, meals and meal times, resting heart rate, and quality of sleep. They were required to turn this in every Monday morning so that adjustments could be made in the subsequent week's cycle of training. Remember that overtraining does not happen overnight. It is a gradual process. Therefore, if the early stages can be recognized, the causal factors can be eliminated and the overtraining prevented.

Breaking the Cycle

To return to the analogy I opened with, in overtraining, the athlete has essentially gone over the edge — he or she has trained too hard for too long. Returning from overtraining is a major rescue operation. Reversing overtraining involves more than rest. It requires recognizing and changing the patterns of an addictive lifestyle. In this case, the addiction is training and competition. Complete rest for a period of time based on the severity of the overtrained state is usually a starting point. There is no set formula for the length of time required for a recovery. It is very individual, based on the factors that made the athlete overtrained and the severity of the overtraining.

Note, however, that with the athlete who is accustomed to a high level of activity (as most overtrained athletes are), complete rest can be a negative shock to the system. Therefore, "active rest," consisting of a low level of activity, would probably be a better alternative. This should be a significant change from normal training activities and of very low intensity. It should be carefully designed to provide just enough stimulus for normal appetite and sleep.

Nutritional therapy is also advised. Generally, this simply involves adjusting the athlete's protein or carbohydrate intake, depending on the type of overtraining. There are various schools of thought about mega-doses of vitamin therapy. Consultation with a nutritionist who has experience working with athletes is recommended. Medical intervention may also be warranted, especially if an iron deficiency is present or the athlete develops an illness, such as mononucleosis.

Psychological counseling may also be necessary, especially if the overtraining is part of an addictive pattern of behaviors. Intervention that is as simple as proper goal setting and relaxation training has proven useful.

It serves to be repeated that overtraining can be a very serious problem and should not be treated with a cavalier attitude. Spot the signs early and stop it before it claims the athlete's competitive season and impairs his or her overall health.

Table Two: What Causes Overtraining?

Many factors can cause overtraining. Following is a list of some of the major factors. It is important to consider the relationship among all of these variables. They are not independent—seldom is one in isolation the cause of the overtraining.

Abuse of toxic substances, especially alcohol: This is especially a problem in certain sports where post-game and post-practice alcohol consumption is part of the culture of the sport.

Loss of weight and extreme fluctuations in weight: For sports like wrestling, gymnastics, boxing, weightlifting, and even running, the effect of constantly having to make weight to stay in a weight class or to strive for a certain appearance to please the judges can exacerbate the process of overtraining.

Lifestyle coupled with hard training: This is especially true for the student who has to stay up late every night studying or who must work a part-time job. Repetitive travel, especially through multiple time zones, also can be especially detrimental.

Poor nutrition: Often, an inadequate or inappropriate diet for the type of training leads to overtraining. The diet might be too low or too high in carbohydrates, or lack enough protein or other essential nutrients. It could also be a poorly designed vegetarian or fad diet. Iron deficiency as a result of an unbalanced diet is a common contributor. Intra-workout nutrition is often neglected, especially hydration.

Neglect of recovery: Both intra-workout and inter-workout recovery is essential. Different systems of the body recover and adapt at different rates — this must be taken into consideration.

Heavily biased workloads, especially a repetition of biased workouts: Workouts that continue to stress one component cause a stagnation, which results in overtraining.

Monotony in training: Doing the same thing every day at the same time in the same sequence will eventually take a severe mental toll.

Poor planning: This encompasses the whole gamut from planning workouts to competition to recovery.

Too much competition: Not having adequate recovery between competitions has deleterious effects, particularly in relation to the athlete's level of development. For the mature, elite athlete, this is less of a problem than for the developing athlete. For example, it is not uncommon in youth sports to have three games during a week and a tournament on a weekend. That is too much — it does not allow for adequate recovery or time for training.

Too fast a rise in intensity or volume of training: Too much too soon does not allow the body to adapt to the stress of training.

The Middle Years — High School

With so many young people involved in sports today, this stage of athletic progress is of great concern to coaches, sport administrators, and parents. My comments in this article are based on my observations from working with athletes and teams at this level, as well as being a parent of a developmental athlete.

What is a developmental athlete? The developmental athlete is one who has gone through the basics of training for his or her respective sport(s) and is beginning to compete at a higher level. It is the middle of three stages of athletic development (See Table One), thus it is also a transitional stage. Another good way to think about it is to consider it the "Training to Compete" phase of development, in which the focus shifts toward preparation for competition and actual competition rather than training to train, which was the emphasis in the previous phase.

The developmental stage encompasses the high school and early college years. In terms of chronological age it spans the ages of 14-20 for boys and 12-18 for girls.

There are several key issues, considerations, and concepts to be discussed relative to this stage of athletic development:

Chronological & Training Age — Traditionally, much of our competition system has been based on chronological, as opposed to developmental age. However, it is unrealistic to expect progress at the same rate and level for all children. In the early years of the developmental phase there are tremendous differences between individuals in terms of maturation, both physically and psychologically. Reliance on chronological age leads to faulty evaluations of potential as well as incorrect training.

Instead, developmental-age athletes need to be judged on a more individual basis, taking into account past progress and current maturity. This is especially important in determining the application of heavy external loads, particularly stress on the spine.

Gender Differences — Because girls mature at a younger age than boys, training demands can often be accelerated for the female athlete, provided there has been a good foundation during the earlier "Training to Train" phase. And with more opportunities for participation for girls, there is also the responsibility to train them for competition.

One very important aspect of training females of this age group is the prevention of ACL injuries. Because there is a higher incidence among girls than boys of this injury, we need to focus on how training may contribute to this trend. I believe the high rate of female ACL injuries is based primarily on the fact that girls tend to train less in the off-season while boys are playing recreational sports, girls often remain inactive when not directly training with their athletic team. They also tend to be less involved in weight training.

Therefore, implementing proper functional strength training and overall preparation to play is critical for female athletes. For this gender, strength training should be performed throughout the training year.

Early Dropout — The developmental period is a stage where there is a high rate of attrition, and much of this is linked to improper emphasis during sports participation. Many young people leave sports because of a poor learning environment, unrealistic expectations placed upon them, and too much intense competition at an early age.

Instead, the early developmental-stage experience should emphasize the basics and provide a sound foundation for further progress. This experience serves to maintain interest, raise motivation, and promote continued participation in sport. The emphasis must be multi-faceted, emphasizing psychological considerations, competition, talent identification, training, and proper coaching/teaching.

The Role of Competition — The key to developing the athlete at any stage is control of the competition schedule. The ultimate goal of training is preparation for competition, but the competition schedule must be closely linked to training. There are three points to consider here: the coach's approach to competition, the ratio of training to competition, and the length of the competitive season.

How competition is approached is very important. Above all, competition should serve as feedback on training progress. The goal should be for each young athlete to strive to better his or her performance measured against his or her previous best. Athletes must experience some degree of success measured against their own standards in order to feel comfortable and to maintain motivation. Early competition in itself is not negative, but it becomes a negative when too much importance is placed upon the result.

Determining an optimal ratio between training and competition is key to ensuring steady progress. In today's environment, the developmental athlete almost has too many competitive opportunities. For the multi-sport athlete, there is competition in some form year-round.

Training athletes during their high school years involves understanding the many factors related to this stage of development.

Even if the athlete specializes, the trend is toward more competitions and multi-seasonal opportunities.

During the early developmental years, the ratio of training to competition should remain high, somewhere in the range of five or six training sessions to one competition. The ratio should shift to three or four to one as the athlete progresses. Competition will assume more of a role as skill and conditioning advance. Remember that competition should serve mainly as feedback to measure progress, as well as to test limits.

Also understand that competition is the highest form of training stress. A rule of thumb is that one competition is equal to at least two hard training sessions in terms of physical and psychological demands.

A final problem with competition at the developmental level is the length of the season. For many highly motivated athletes, there is never an off-season where they can just train. For example, in soccer, the combined club season, high school season, and ODP program begins in late August and continues to early July. Basketball, volleyball, and to a certain extent, football are also becoming year-round competitive sports. The athletes have less and less time to recharge their batteries.

Talent Identification and Direction — The fundamental assumption is that if talent is identified early, nurtured, and developed to its fullest extent, gifted athletes will continue on to the highest levels of competition. However, in the United States, we have traditionally taken a different approach. The assumption here is that if a large, healthy population base is available, then a process based on competition and letting the strong survive allows the best athletes to surface. This system has traditionally worked well for the US. However, as other nations take a more systematic approach to the nurturing of young athletes, we may be falling behind.

The model utilized by the former GDR (East Germany) is a successful example of a system based on talent identification and direction. That system entailed a gradual progression that continually worked to select and match young athletes to events or sports that were suited to their body types and abilities. The emphasis was on the development of general athletic qualities as a foundation for later specialization. The philosophy was that training must progress over a six- to ten-year period to achieve top results, and that through this planned progression, ultimate success would come in the adult years. The program was closely tied to the educational system through mandatory physical education taught by highly trained specialists. While this might not be appropriate in the US, it is an interesting method that should continue to be examined.

Specialization vs. the Multi-Sport Athlete — A danger of early identification of talent is the narrowing of skills through early specialization in one sport or event. This can easily occur if the initial identification of talent is based on a dominant physical characteristic such as size, speed, or strength biased by accelerated growth and/or maturation. Early specialization can also predispose young athletes to injury either from overuse or growth-plate damage due to improper loading.

The first time specialization should begin is during the early developmental phase. However, this specialization should still be fairly broad. For example, it can be in a sport rather than a specific position or event. In track and field the specialization would be in the throwing events; later specialization would be in only one of the throws. In team sports, it is preferable to have the athlete play a variety of positions before specializing in one position. At the other end of the spectrum, a common problem for the multi-sport athlete is juggling the training between two or three sports. It has been my experience that the best way to handle the situation is to use the athlete's strength training as the unifying element.

Another problem is handling the transition time when the multi-sport athlete switches seasons between sports. Due to the short seasons in most high school sports, it is unrealistic for the athlete to take two weeks without competition to make the transition. Only the cooperation of all the involved coaches can ensure that the athlete does not get caught in a training tug-of-war.

Training — For the developmental athlete, the acquisition of motor skills relates more to maturity and the learning process than any other variables. Remember, children are not miniature adults, and their biomotor abilities must be developed in an appropriate manner. As stated by Piscopo and Baley in *Kinesiology-The Science of Movement*, "Optimum motor learning develops in children when skills are taught at the right time (maturation-readiness) and in the proper manner (experience-practices)."

The crucial years for motor learning are the so-called "Skill Hungry" years from ages seven to nine. This is when fundamental motor skills should be taught to provide a foundation for more specialized skills that will follow at an older age. Strength and endurance will increase with growth and maturity. Thus, big muscle skills should follow fine motor skills.

Effective training for the beginning developmental athlete should encompass all of the following: 1) proper conditioning; 2) good, competent coaching; 3) grouping according to skill, body size, and physical maturation; 4) safe equipment; and 5) rules and equipment modified to meet the athletes' physical limitations and skills.

Let's also not forget the most fundamental principle of training: progression. Proper progression throughout a training year and throughout a career should encompass the following: basic conditioning, basic technical model, specific advanced conditioning, and advanced technical model. On a smaller level, first increase the frequency of the workouts, then increase the duration of the workouts, and finally, increase the demands of the training.

The developmental phase is just one stage in the progress of an athlete, but it is an important one. If we can train our pre-teens and teenagers in the proper methods, we can come that much closer to having a healthy adult population with appropriate skills and ideas on athletics.

Table One: Three Periods of Development

Foundation Period: Training To Train
- Begins in a range from 9 to 11 years
- Three to four years in duration
- Games and fun activities, wide variety designed to enhance self-image
- General training, speed development, motor skill development
- Develop bodyweight strength, mobility, and aerobic endurance
- Develop basic skills and rhythm
- One training session per week increasing to three per week
- Competition should be limited and confined to playful situations

Developmental Period: Training To Compete
- Begins in a range from 13 to 14 years for males and 12 to 13 years for girls
- Four to six years in duration
- Emphasize general training in the first years
- Amount of specific training should increase gradually over the last two years
- Develop appropriate training and competition behavior
- Begin goal setting appropriate to level of development
- Teach weight training techniques with submaximal loading
- Three training sessions per week increasing to six in later years
- Undertake formal competition, which should increase in difficulty as the athlete advances through the developmental period

Period of Mature Participation: Training To Win
- Begins in a range from 17 to 22 years
- Not before 17 or after 22
- Percentage of specific training sessions increases
- The time spent within the training sessions increases significantly, especially for the elite athlete
- Competition frequency and difficulty increases significantly

References:
Bales, J., "Lessons from the GRD," *Coaching Review*, Sept./Oct., 1986, p. 30-32.

Brook, N.D., "Conditioning and the Growing Athlete," *Athletics Coach*, Vol. 19, No. 4, Dec., 1985, p. 31-35.

Piscopo, J., and Bailey, J.A., *Kinesiology — The Science of Movement*, John Wiley & Sons, New York, 1981, p. 152.

Measure For Measure

Regardless of one's specific training philosophy and methods, testing and evaluation should be an integral part of the training process. Many coaches treat testing as a separate component or implement it sporadically. However, if an athlete is to be successful in achieving his or her goals, testing must work in concert with the overall strength and conditioning program.

Because the training process consists of incremental gains in pursuit of a special goal, it is important to ascertain how much progress toward that goal is being achieved. The best way to accomplish this is to periodically assess the training status of the athlete. It is for this reason that testing and evaluation should be viewed as an essential feedback mechanism in the training process — not as a separate component.

The purpose of testing is, initially, to gather baseline data on general physical parameters such as speed, strength, power, endurance, as well as the biomechanical and physiological status of the athlete. This will help determine the athlete's strengths and weaknesses relative to the demands of the athlete's particular sport and assist in determining what activities will optimize training.

After the initial assessment, testing is then used to measure progress from training period to training period or from year to year. Periodic testing will also provide information to predict performance as well as to plan for peak performance.

Testing can also be used to compare an athlete to other athletes on the team or to past athletes at similar stages in their careers. This can be a tremendous aid in goal setting and positive motivation for the athlete.

Types of Tests

Testing may take several different forms, depending on your goals. Consider the following:

Criteria tests identify a specific biomotor quality. The criteria test is usually administered once or twice during a training year and should represent the athlete's best effort.

Progress checks are administered periodically to assess the progress of training relative to the training goal.

There are times in a training program when an indicator workout can be more valuable than testing. This is especially true with athletes that you have been training for a number of years. An annual indicator workout conducted under controlled conditions will allow the athlete and coach to accurately assess progress in pursuit of a specific goal. The results can be compared to previous years' results to indicate progress or lack of progress.

For most sport situations, field tests are preferable to lab tests. Results from field tests are simply much more practical and realistic than those from lab tests, because field tests are conducted under conditions which are much closer to actual competition. They also allow the coach to be a key part of the testing process, which makes it more personal for the athlete.

If you have the facilities and the time to use laboratory tests, they can be useful to periodically establish baseline measures. This is especially true for invasive physiological testing and biomechanical analysis. The key to lab testing is for the coach to receive help in interpreting the results and applying them to the objectives of the training. The competition or game analysis is an often overlooked aspect of the testing process. A win or an improved performance is often considered a successful competition, while a loss or a poor performance is considered a failure. However, competitions should be analyzed—disregarding the final score — and used to evaluate and revise the training plan (See Table One).

By regularly testing your athletes, you can assess the effectiveness of your training program and provide motivation for your athletes.

Table One: Competition Analysis

Day/Date: Time of Day: (Be specific)

Opponent: Climate/Weather Conditions: (Be specific)

Warm-up: Was it a regular warm-up? Was it interrupted?

Actual Competition Analysis: How was the performance relative to the stage of training and the competition? Where are you in relation to your goals?

Recommendations for the Future: How can I learn from this competition? What would I do differently?

Changes Needed in Training: How can or do I need to modify training based on the competition result? How do any changes reconcile with the training plan?

Table Two

Serial test results of University of Illinois hurdler Dawn Riley

	92-93	93-94	94-95	95-96
Standing Long Jump	2.65 m	2.80 m	2.76 m	2.81 m
Standing Triple Jump	7.65 m	8.18 m	8.19 m	8.33 m
30-meter Fly	3.57 sec	3.29 sec	3.39 sec	3.30 sec
55-meter Hurdles	7.81 sec	7.76 sec	7.76 sec	7.60 sec
Squat	No Test	No Test	145 Kg	170 Kg
Clean	No Test	No Test	75 Kg	80 Kg
100-meter Hurdles	13.85 sec	13.62 sec	13.36 sec	No Test
200 meters	25.02 sec	24.22 sec	23.78 sec	23.95 sec
300 meters	43.27 sec	No Test	39.17 sec	38.96 sec

Looking at Results

For the individual athlete, it is important to stress individual improvement in performance relative to previous test results (See Table Two.). If results show unexpected drops in performance, training can be adjusted. When results show progress, it reinforces to the athlete the benefits of his or her hard work.

As your testing program progresses, it will enable the development of sport/event-specific and population-specific norms. Once you have tested a group of athletes at least four times, it is then possible to develop norms to use in comparing those athletes within that training group. Obviously, the more test data that is gathered on that particular group, the more valid the information will be.

It is helpful to establish mean values for each represented event or position, as well as mean values for the entire training group. To rank athletes, the best method is to use standard deviation from the mean (See Table Three). For motivational purposes, I have also found it valuable to compare the group testing averages in the beginning of the season from year to year (See Table Four).

For the coach, it can be helpful to compare one athlete's results against the group results in order to see if there are any trends. For example, if one or two individuals increase their vertical jump beyond their teammates' while on a special training program, then it would be advisable to re examine the training of the whole group.

Administering Testing

For testing to be worthwhile, it must meet the standards of validity and reliability. To be valid the test must measure what it is intended to test. Reliability means it must consistently measure a given factor. To accomplish this, the tests must be administered in exactly the same way each time, and, if at all possible, by the same person.

For testing to be motivational but non-threatening to the athlete, the athlete should understand the philosophy and meaning of each of the individual tests. He or she must also understand that test results measure and guide progress, but are not a major factor in team selection — that the ultimate test of performance is in the arena of competition.

Tests must also be easily administered and interpreted. The instruction and the expected outcome should be simple and clear to both the test administrator and the athlete. If the requirements of the test are not easily interpreted, then the athlete will end up concentrating on the test, rather than on his or her performance, yielding very unreliable results. It follows that the tests should not require much equipment.

Table Three: Test Score Rating for Speed/Power Sports

	10 Yard Burst	40 Yard Sprint	Verticle Jump	30 Sec Cone Jump
Superior	<1.30	< 4.55	30 or >	60 or >
Excellent	1.31-1.40	4.56-4.79	28-29	58-59
Good	1.41-1.50	4.80-4.90	25-27	55-57
Average	1.51-1.60	4.91-5.10	23-24	53-54
Poor	≥1.61	≥ 5.11	≤ 22	≤ 52

*All times are measured electronically.

Also, be sure to allow adequate recovery time between individual tests. For very demanding tests, such as the criteria test, make sure the athlete is well rested and prepared before the test in order to show peak results. It is helpful to take the viewpoint that testing represents the highest quality effort short of actual competition.

Although not a formal part of the testing process, daily quantification (when coordinated with testing information) can provide valuable feedback. Such daily record keeping should begin early in the athlete's career to provide a chronological overview of training progress. This should be the responsibility of the athlete as well as the coach. The goal is to record every workout and be as detailed as possible. Then, if a weakness appears in the results of a test, you already know what training has or has not been done to address it.

Test Examples
Speed Tests
Ten Yard Burst — from a sport specific starting position. To test starting ability.

Sprint — 20, 30, 40, 50, 60, 75 yards. To test acceleration.

Flying start — 20, 30, 40, 50 yards to test absolute (top end) speed.

Agility Tests
Ski Hex Jump — To test body control. Suitable for all sports as a test of body awareness, control, and coordination.

Agility 5-10-5 — To test change of direction.

T Test — A test of combinations of movements. Commonly used in basketball, tennis, soccer, and baseball.

Nebraska Agility — A test of combinations of movements. This is commonly used in football.

Pro Shuttle—A basic progressive change-of-direction test.

Table Four: Professional Team Training Camp Test Averages

1992 Training Camp Testing

	Best	Worst	Average	Standard Deviation
Flexibility	24	14	19	2.5
Vertical Jump	30.5	19.5	24.43	2.24
Quick Feet	131	86	111	11.64
Standing Long Jump	118	86	103.4	6.81
30 Sec Cone Jump	69	45	59.22	4.50
Agility	8.36	10.9	9.15	0.34
Ten Yard Burst	1.60	1.99	1.77	0.17
Medicine Ball Throw	78	50	60.15	7.50
300 yd. Shuttle	52.58	62.36	55.87	1.86

1993 Training Camp Testing

	Best	Worst	Average	Standard Deviation
Flexibility	26	14	20	2.3
Vertical Jump	38.5	21.5	27.92	3.57
Quick Feet	139	84	116	10.64
Standing Long Jump	129	88	106.4	7.4
30 Sec Cone Jump	70	51	59.4	3.7
Agility	8.20	9.97	9.10	0.32
Ten Yard Burst	1.58	1.98	1.72	0.07
Medicine Ball Throw	82	48	61.15	7.24
300 yd. Shuttle	50.91	59.85	54.97	2.01

Myrland Star Test — A test to determine the athlete's ability to move to the right and compare movement to the left based on the wheel principle.

Anaerobic Power and Capacity Tests

300 Yard Shuttle — 25 yards in length. Six times down and back. Five minutes recovery before a second run. The score is the average time of the two runs.

45 Second All-out Run for Distance — Measure total distance run in 45 sec to the nearest meter.

Margaria Stair Test — A test of power calculated from the time required to run a predetermined distance up a staircase.

30-Second Wingate Test — A test of anaerobic power done on a friction bike.

60-Second Vertical Jump Test

Aerobic Power and Capacity Tests

Treadmill Max Test

Legér Test — This is a multi-stage test in which the athlete runs back and forth over a 20-meter distance at predetermined paces based on an auditory tone. This is sometimes called a beep test.

Cooper Test — A run on a track to see how much distance can be covered in twelve minutes.

Power Tests

Vertical Jump — Also known as the sergeant jump. The athlete crouches down and then jumps up as high as possible. The height of the jump is determined by the difference between standing reach and the reach during the jump.

Step/Close Jump — The same as the vertical jump with the addition of a step.

Standing Long Jump — With a two-foot takeoff, jump out as far as possible.

Standing Triple Jump — From a standing position, hop, skip, and jump as far as possible.

Three- or Five-repeat Standing Long Jumps — the same as the standing long jump but repeated three or five times consecutively.

30-Second Cone Jump — The athlete jumps side to side over 12-inch cones.

Overback Medicine Ball Throw — The athlete swings the ball down between the legs and throws the ball over the back while extending the legs and the trunk.

Forward through-the-legs Medicine Ball Throw — The athlete swings the ball down between the legs and throws it forward while extending the legs and the trunk.

Seated Medicine Ball Throw — Seated with the back firmly against a chair, the athlete throws the ball out as far as possible using a chest-pass motion.

Anthropometric Tests

Body Composition

Six or Seven Site Skinfolds

Hydrostatic Weighing

Photo — Front and Side View (before and after training)

Limb Length and Body Dimensions

Nutritional Assessment — Usually based on a three- or five-day diet scan in which all nutrients are analyzed.

There are a myriad of tests available and the above are only a sampling. The key is to select the tests that fit with the sport that you are coaching and the athlete population that is participating in that particular sport. Make sure the tests have a specific purpose that fits into the overall plan.

For a detailed description of many of the tests mentioned see: *Physiological Testing of the High Performance Athlete* (Second Edition), MacDougal, Wenger, and Green editors. Published by Human Kinetics Books, Champaign, Illinois. ◆

Evaluating Training

Think back to your school days. Whether it was high school, college, or grade school, we were all taught similar subjects and progressed through the system by meeting certain standards. Along the way, progress was continually evaluated through tests.

Now, use the same model for your athletes. Consider every competition a big exam. For them to succeed, you must train their abilities. But you probably won't be able to do that optimally without continually testing them along the way and identifying and correcting any weaknesses.

One of our biggest responsibilities as coaches is to find the most effective manner to evaluate our athletes' efforts and progress in training, as well as in competition. A good, sound assessment program will provide needed guidance and direction to make training as meaningful as possible.

Testing = Training

Testing and training go together like hand and glove. Evaluation through testing is an ongoing process that will determine the direction and content of training. Therefore, it is important to build testing into every stage of the training plan.

The traditional approach has been to schedule specific days for testing, usually at the beginning or the end of a yearly training cycle. This usually consists of criteria tests that profile the athlete with respect to the biomotor requirements of a particular sport.

Over the past several years I have grown increasingly uncomfortable with this approach. Testing only twice in a yearly cycle gave me good baseline information, but it did not provide much insight about the athlete's ongoing progress. Yet this information is crucial in making day-to-day and week-to-week adjustments in the athlete's training to obtain optimum adaptive response.

As I began to work with an increasing variety of sports, I quickly saw the need to incorporate day-to-day testing into the actual training process. While this may seem a bit extreme, I assure that you can continually test your athletes while still training them, and not overwhelm them.

The solution is to follow the concept that "testing equals training and training equals testing." You don't need to stop each athlete every few minutes and run him or her through a battery of tests. At various points in each training session, there are distinct windows of opportunity to get feedback as to the effects of training. It is imperative to take advantage of these periods to look for this feedback (his or her response to a given component of training) and utilize it to plan ongoing training.

Continually testing your athletes' performance will enable you to better customize their training.

Training is cumulative, so it is important to keep the big picture in mind. Ongoing evaluation enables us to keep everything in proportion and perspective. The challenge is to make testing meaningful to all concerned—athletes, coaches, and medical support staff. You are testing for feedback and verification that the training is achieving the desired results.

When you are testing, it is important to consider all of the following:

Know what you are looking for. There are periods of training where you should see marked improvement and other times when you should see stabilization or even slight regression on certain tests. Remember, the tests should reflect the training.

- Know what you are going to do when you find it. If you see regression, what adjustments will you make? Conversely, if you see unexpected improvement, what will you do?
- Testing helps to individualize training. There is much individual variability in adaptive responses to different training stimuli. Two individuals could have the opposite response to the same training session or training cycle. Testing can identify how each individual will respond and allow training adjustments to be made accordingly.
- Testing will give constant feedback to the athletes and coaches as to the effects of training. Do not wait until competition to ascertain training response; be proactive by regularly testing. Testing must dovetail into training. It is an integral part of the whole training spectrum. It is important to remember that the goal of testing is to determine each individual player's athletic qualities relative to the demands of his or her position and the game. I am not interested in comparing an athlete against some arbitrary norms, but I am interested in intra-individual comparison: comparing him or her against him- or herself.
- Test what you are training! If you are in power phase, your tests should reflect the emphasis on power training.
- Assess progress toward a goal. This also enables you to set realistic goals and adjust the goals accordingly.

Do not use testing to:
- Select a team. Team selection should be based on results in the competitive arena of the actual sport. Tests can verify what you see or do not see during competition, but they should not be the sole criteria for team selection.

- Predict performance. Testing can be used as a status report on progress toward a goal. But performance in the actual game, match, or meet is dependent on so much more than the physical capacities identified through testing.

The criteria for any test is that it must be:
- Reliable. The same results must be obtained each time no matter who is doing the testing.
- Valid. The tests must measure what they purport to measure. For example, a speed test must be a test of speed not speed endurance.
- Practical. The test must be easy to administer and interpret. It must yield information that the coach and athlete can understand and use, or it becomes testing for testing sake. Do not have so many tests that you gather more information than you can use. This will confuse all involved.

A Multitude of Tests

There are a wide variety of tests that satisfy these criteria. One of the most important is biomechanical assessment. This used to be outside the realm of possibility for most people, but with the availability of digital cameras and simple analysis programs, biomechanical assessment is now a viable option at any level of performance.

Assessment of each athlete's biomechanics is something that should be done during workout and competition to establish baseline measures. Then you can continually compare to that baseline. It does not have to be extremely sophisticated to provide very good information.

The "test set" concept from swimming is another excellent tool to assess current training status. This simply means that you have certain indicator workouts that are interspersed throughout the training year that are indicative of the athlete's training progress in pursuit of a specific goal.

In addition to the baseline information and training progress, it is also important to always know how far the athlete is off of his or her best performance level. For example, in the special preparation phase with my 400-meter runners, I like to use a six-minute continuous hill workout progressing to 2 x 6 minutes of hills with three minutes rest. The goal is to see how many hills each sprinter can run in six minutes and to see if he or she can match that number in the second six-minute set. This workout gives me a good reading on each athlete's ability to handle more intense work of a special endurance nature.

At different times in the training year, how much variation between an athlete's current performance and his or her best performance is acceptable? I follow the guide of Gennadi Touretski, the coach of Alexander Popov, world record holder in the 100-meter freestyle. Gennadi feels that at anytime in the training year, Popov should not be further than ten percent off of his best performance. To ensure this, periodic testing is incorporated throughout the training program.

Fitting It All In

The simplest way to incorporate testing often while still training your athletes is to buy into the concept that "testing equals training and training equals testing." Thus, when conducting assessments, the best place to start the process is with the warm-up. This is your first opportunity each day to evaluate the effects of yesterday's workout, as well as the athlete's preparedness for today's workout. Include tasks that test the athlete's balance and coordination. This will offer good feedback as to the athlete's state of readiness. And have alternate or contingency plans available based on what you observe during the warm-up.

One must also learn to time and measure everything that is reasonable to measure during a practice. Dean Smith, former men's basketball coach at the University of North Carolina, made use of this throughout his coaching career. He quantified everything in practice. If he was running athletes through a shooting drill, he kept track of every shot made versus missed, and he made sure each athlete was aware of his stats. The UNC women's soccer team adopted this concept with great success.

In sports like swimming and track and field, which are much more quantifiable, timing and measuring can be incorporated on a day-to-day basis even easier than in sports like soccer and basketball. Essentially, it is good record-keeping that enables you, the coaches, and the athletes to know where things stand at all times.

While acknowledging the important role of testing, we must be careful not to draw too many conclusions from one series of tests. Only after several tests have been conducted periodically throughout the training year can an in-depth profile of each athlete be determined. In most instances, the tests will indicate deficiencies that were already identified through observation of training and game performance. But they serve to further pinpoint those deficiencies. Tests give specific numbers to compare for improvement and motivation. But remember, the ultimate test is the actual competition.

Interpreting the Test Results

Athlete: Professional soccer player (forward)
Phase of Training: During training camp (preseason)

> *I am not interested in comparing an athlete against some arbitrary norms, but I am interested in intra-individual comparison — comparing him or her against him- or herself.*

Purpose of Tests: This battery of tests was used to evaluate starting ability, core and leg strength, explosive power, and power endurance. All tests were electronically timed to ensure accuracy.

10-Meter Start
The athlete should use a standing start off the right foot, then repeat starting off the left foot (indicates which foot is forward). This tests the athlete's ability to accelerate. A deficiency here indicates a lack of strength and/or poor starting technique. It would be best if there were as little difference as possible between the two times. That would indicate symmetry starting off both legs, which is desirable in soccer.

20-Meter Flying Start
Have the athlete begin running twenty meters back from the start to ensure that he or she is at top speed during the 20-meter test distance. This indicates top-end speed. This is also used to indicate closing speed as expressed in meters per second. This is how much distance a player can cover in a particular time. A deficiency here indicates a lack of speed due to lack of power (also indicated on repetitive jump test) or poor acceleration technique.

50-Meter "Ajax" Shuttle
Set two lines ten meters apart. The player begins at line A, then runs and touches line B, plants, and returns to line A. Have him or her repeat this five times for a total of 50 meters. This test indicates the ability to start, stop, and restart. A deficiency here indicates a lack of functional leg strength and core strength. For an athlete at this player's level, a score under 10 seconds is considered very good.

Bengsbo "Intermittent-Recovery" Beep Test
This is a 20-meter multi-stage shuttle test. Set two lines 20 meters apart. On your auditory signal, the athlete runs from one line to the other. The time between signals gets progressively quicker, so that the athlete can easily make it from one line to the other in the span between the first two signals, but by the 40th or so signal, he or she will have trouble making it in time. This test assesses specific endurance in terms of the utilization of oxygen. A deficiency here indicates a lack of overall work capacity. One thousand meters is considered the minimum standard to be able to play 90 minutes at the highest levels.

Jump Test — Squat Jump
Have the athlete start in a stationary squat position with the thighs parallel to the floor. This tests the contractile properties of the muscles, which relates to the standing start.

Jump Test Counter-Movement Jump
The athlete should start in a standing position and quickly squat down and jump as high as possible. This tests the elastic properties of muscle, or basic explosive power. Performance on this test relates to the 20-Meter Fly. It would be best to see a significant difference between the height on the squat jump and the counter-movement jump.

Jump Test — Repetitive Jump
Have the athlete perform as many counter-movement jumps as possible in 15 seconds. This tests power and power endurance. Performance on this test also relates to the 20-Meter Fly.

The following are specific training recommendations based on all test results:
10-Meter Left
Best: 1.83 sec   Average: 1.86 sec   Range: 0.6 sec
10-Meter Right
Best: 1.77 sec   Average: 1.80 sec   Range: 0.7 sec
20-Meter Fly
Best: 2.45 sec   Average: 2.48 sec   Range: 0.5 sec
Maximum Velocity m/s: 8.16
Illinois Agility
Best: 16.00 sec   Average: 16.05 sec   Range: 0.1 sec
Ajax Shuttle
Best: 10.73 sec   Average: 10.79 sec   Range: 0.6 sec
Beep Test
Distance: 920 meters
Squat Jump
Height: 0.464 meters
Counter-Movement Jump
Height: 0.484 meters
Repetitive Jump
Number of Jumps: 15 Average Height: 0.414 meters
Power: 31.16 w/kg

Evaluation: His jump tests indicate good power potential, but it does not show up in the speed and agility tests. Also, this athlete tends to take too long a first step. These traits are reflected on the field in his inability to gain a step on the opposition.

Thus, acceleration work should be practiced twice a week, with drills involving short bursts with an emphasis on good technique. Work agility the same day as acceleration. Here, the emphasis should be on quick change of direction and footwork. But ultimately, this athlete should be doing some agility work each day! ◆

Regeneration Gap

As we strive to push our athletes toward better and better performances, we usually focus on altering their workload—the microcycles, sessions, sets and reps, and so forth. However, it may be just as important to focus on the athlete's recovery. The more that I analyze my past coaching successes and failures as well as examining other programs, the more I realize that the key to success is not the work, but the rest.

How many times have you heard of an athlete incurring a minor injury, missing a week of training, then coming back to record a lifetime best in a subsequent competition? Everyone marvels at this, the usual comment being, "Just think what would have happened if she had not missed that week of training." The reality of the situation, however, was that the athlete was probably training too hard, and the injury gave her a chance to recover. In fact, had she continued to train, she probably would not have performed as well.

This explanation seems like a contradiction until you begin to understand the process of training and recovery. Training is the application of stress and subsequent adaptation during the recovery period. When you look at that statement closely, you'll see that adaptation is half the formula. It follows that, if the body is not given the proper recovery, it simply will not adapt to the stress— and progress will not occur.

In the United States, we tend to overlook the role of recovery in the training process. Traditionally, we take a reactive approach, attempting to rehab overtraining or overuse injuries after they occur. However, I've started to take a closer look at systematic approaches to recovery and regeneration used by coaches in other countries, and have begun to pay more attention to this important aspect of training with my own athletes. The approach is very proactive, and the goal is simple: to optimize the training process. In this article, I will share some of the things that I have learned on this important topic, along with some practical suggestions for incorporating restoration techniques into your training.

The Basics
In order to clarify the concept and ensure consistent terminology, I'll start by defining and explaining the basic terms.

Rest is time off with no training at all. For the highly competitive athlete, rest is rarely a good choice. When an athlete is accustomed to the stress of training, no activity at all is a negative shock to the system.

Recovery and regeneration is often thought of as something that occurs when you're not training. It's time to, instead, see it as an integral part of training.

Active Rest is time when muscles work, but nerves rest. It is time off from the regular activities of training, but not time off from activity. It often involves other sports or physical activities. Active rest is preferable to complete rest.

Restoration consists of activities or external means (e.g., massage) that help the athlete to physically or psychologically overcome the rigors of hard training and bring his or her energy back to a baseline level or higher. Restoration is an active, not passive, process.

Recovery is an actual planned unit in the training schedule. Its goal is to return the athlete to previous performance levels.

Planning Recovery
The most common approach to developing a training plan is to determine and schedule the workload, with recovery as an afterthought. However, over the years, I have found this approach often leads to a big difference between work planned and work accomplished. Athletes do not recover properly and, as a result, are unable to finish workouts (or they complete workouts in a less than satisfactory manner). This is both physically and psychologically defeating.

Workout plans should, instead, start with the recovery, followed by the work. I have found that taking this approach allows me to be much more exact in planning workloads, and I get more out of the athletes because they are recovered and able to handle a greater workload. The ability to recover should dictate the volume and intensity of the workouts, not the other way around.

In order to plan recovery we need to first answer two questions: **How do I know when recovery has occurred?** Basically, recovery occurs when the athlete's energy stores are replenished. Any residual soreness from previous workouts should subside after warm-up, and the body language of the athlete is lively. Mentally, the athlete wants to do the work—he or she does not have to get "psyched."

How long does it take to recover? This is a more difficult question to answer, as it depends on the type of work being done, as well as the individual's ability to recover from that work.

The first factor to consider is the sport. If the sport is non-weightbearing, like swimming, rowing, or cycling, it has less of an eccentric component, and athletes can handle a greater volume of work and still recover quickly. However, athletes in weightbearing sports will need longer recovery periods. For example, a runner or a basketball player cannot handle as great a workload as a swimmer, because these sports involve a heavier load of eccentric work.

Also take a look at the characteristics of the sport and determine if it is contact, collision, or non-contact. Contact sports like basketball and soccer require a fairly long recovery period because of the physical contact coupled with the aerobic demand. Collision sports like football and rugby need even longer recovery times to allow healing to occur.

Perhaps the toughest aspect of planning recovery time is that there are individual differences to consider. Just as each athlete has a different capacity to tolerate the stress of training, each athlete has a different rate of recovery.

One major factor that contributes to this difference is the athlete's state of fitness. In general, the higher the athlete's overall fitness, the more quickly the athlete will recover between workouts and competitions.

Another easy-to-assess contributor is age. Both chronological and training age are significant factors in recovery. The masters athlete must allow more time to recover between workouts and competitions than the younger athlete, who generally has the capacity to recover more quickly and to handle a greater workload.

Body type, particularly in regard to body composition, also has an impact on recovery. Leaner, more heavily muscled athletes have a tougher time recovering, especially in contact and collision sports.

Total Training Stress (TTS), the cumulative stress of training and living, is often overlooked as a factor in recovery. However, we need to realize that the athletes we are working with are more a product of what they do the other 19 to 20 hours out of the day than the four or five hours a day devoted to actual training. To optimize recovery, and therefore training, we must carefully consider diet, sleep, work, school, relationships, and so forth. It is safe to make the generalization that lifestyle is the biggest factor in the athlete's ability or inability to recover.

Hastening Recovery

As noted earlier, recovery and regeneration should be active processes. They can be affected by what is done before, during, and after the workout, and by the structure of the workout. We must first consider recovery both intra-workout and inter-workout. Intra-workout refers to recovery within a workout such as rest between sets in weight training or rest between runs in an interval workout. The rest should be "active rest." For example, have athletes stretch between sets during weight training; and they should walk or jog after heavy lactate work. Be sure to also allow adequate time to recover between exercises and the various types of work. In addition, proper nutrition during the workout--fluid and carbohydrate replacement--will improve recovery and enhance the quality of the workout.

Inter-workout recovery refers to recovery between sessions, either between a morning session and an afternoon session, or from day to day. The simplest manifestation of this type of recovery is the so-called Hard/Easy Principle popularized by former University of Oregon track coach Bill Bowerman. His rule, which has stood the test of time, is to always have an easy workout day follow a hard workout day to allow the body to recover. More specifically, do not put two sessions of high neuromuscular-demand work, like sprinting or plyometrics, back-to-back. Instead, follow such work with an easy session of light aerobic exercises and stretching to ensure proper recovery.

Another important way to enhance recovery is to plan complementary work. Certain types of work complement each other, while other types of work contradict. Some examples of complementary work are: speed and strength; strength endurance and endurance; strength and elastic strength; and skill, speed, and elastic strength. The effect of this type of work is synergistic. Conversely, when performing contradictory drills, the effect of one training method detracts from the other training method.

The warm-up and cool down are also critical components of hastening recovery. The warm-up should activate the athletes' muscles slowly. It can include massage, relaxing and stretching, and relaxed free-rhythmic exercises, as well as any light exercise. The cool-down can include any type of low intensity aerobic work, such as light free exercise, relaxation and stretching, and walking. Because the cool down is usually the least favorite part of the workout, playing simple games can keep an athlete properly motivated.

Restoration can also be enhanced by off-the-field physiological methods such as massage, relaxing baths, saunas, and hydrotherapy. Although proper nutrition is a very obvious part of restoration, it cannot be emphasized enough. The athlete's diet should be evaluated for deficiencies, as well as for the rhythm and size of meals. Mental training, such as concentration/relaxation training, can also prove very helpful.

Considering Competitions

Competition of any type provides greater stress than training, thus frequent competition usually requires more recovery. Again, this is dependent on the type of sport, as well as the length of the competitive season in relation to the off-season, and the ratio of workouts to competition. In any case, keep in mind that restoration methods should begin immediately after competition ends, and training should be carefully planned around recovery from competition.

Another consideration with respect to recovery and

competition is preparing for a game/match/meet where there are heats, semifinals, and finals or a tournament situation. In this case, performing two or three hard training sessions back-to-back is advisable to simulate the competitive scenario. It is better to see how the athlete reacts to this type of stress in a controlled situation, rather than in actual competition.

In Closing

Overall, the time before, after, and between workouts and competition should be viewed as a critical part of the training process. Have your athletes experiment with what types of recovery activities work best for them. For some athletes, light jogging for 20 minutes immediately after the workout and massage four hours later may be best. Others may respond better to playing simple games following the workout, a long walk later in the day, and using relaxation methods throughout the day. In any case, incorporating these concepts of recovery and regeneration should allow your athletes ultimately to achieve higher fitness levels. ◆

Suggested Reading

Albert, Mark.(1991) *Eccentric Muscle Training In Sports And Orthopaedics.* New York: Churchill Livingstone.

Bloomfield, J. Ackland, T.R. and Elliot, B.C. Editors. *Applied Anatomy And Biomechanics In Sport*, Carlton, Australia: Blackwell Scientific Publications, 1994.

Bosco, Carmelo. *Stretch-shortening Cycle in Skeletal Muscle Function and Physiological Considerations On Explosive Power in Man, Atleticastudi,#1*, pp. 7-113, 1985.

Chaitow L: *Muscle Energy Techniques.* New York: Churchill Livingstone, 1997.

Curwin, Sandra. & Stanish, William D. M.D. *Tendinitis: it's etiology and treatment*, Lexington, Massachusetts: D.C. Heath and Company, 1984.

Cavanagh, Peter R. Editor. *Biomechanics of Distance Running*, Human Kinetic Books, Champaign, IL., 1990.

Dirix, A., Knuttgen, H.G., and Tittel, K. Editors. *The Olympic Book Of Sports Medicine*, Oxford, England: Blackwell Scientific Publications, 1988.

Drabik, Jo'zef Ph.D., *Children & Sports Training*, Island Pond, Vermont: Stadion Publishing Company, Inc., 1996.

Dominguez, Richard H. M.D., and Gajda, Robert S. (1982) *Total Body Training.* New York, N.Y: Warner Books.

Dorrance, Anson and Averbuch. *The Vision Of A Champion.* Chelsea, MI: Sleeping Bear Press, 2002.

Enoka, Roger M., *Neuromechanical Basis of Kinesiology,* Second Edition. Champaign, Illinois: Human Kinetics Books, Inc. 1994.

Fleck, Steven J., and Kraemer, William J. Second edition(1997) *Designing Resistance Training Programs.* Champaign, Illinois: Human Kinetics Books.

Gabbard, Carl., Leblanc, Elizabeth., and Lowy, Susan. *Physical Education for Children-Building the Foundation*, Englewood Cliffs, New Jersey. Prentice-Hall, Inc. 1987.

Gambetta, Vern. and Odgers, Steve., *The Complete Guide To Medicine Ball Training*, Sarasota, Florida: Optimum Sports Training, 1991.

Grabiner, Mark D. Editor. *Current Issues in Biomechanics*, Champaign, Illinois: Human Kinetics Books Inc., 1993.

Gustavsen R, Streeck R: *Training Therapy; Prophylaxis and Rehabilitation*, New York, Thieme Medical Publishers 1993.

Gray, Gary. (1991) *Dumbbells-R-Smart*, Adrian, MI: Wynn Marketing.

Gray GW: *Chain reaction festival; Course manual*, Chicago, IL 1996.

Hannaford, Carla, *Smart Moves – Why Learning Is Not All In Your Head*, Great Ocean Publishers. Arlington, Virginia 1995.

Ireland, Mary Lloyd, Gaudette, and Cook, Scoot. *ACL Injuries in the Female Athlete, Journal of Sport Rehabilitation*, 1997, vol. 6. Pp. 97 -110.

Jesse J: *Hidden Causes of Injury, Prevention, And Correction for Running Athletes*, The Athletic Press. Pasadena, CA 1977.

Jones, Norman L. et. al. (1986) *Human Muscle Power*, Champaign, IL: Human Kinetics Publishing Company.

Komi, P. V., Editor, *Strength And Power In Sport*, London: Blackwell Scientific Publications1992.

Kurz, Thomas., *Science of Sports Training*, Island Pont, Vt: Stadion Publishing Company, 2001 – Second Edition.

Kurz, Thomas., *Stretching Scientifically – A guide to flexibility training*, Third Edition. Island Pont, Vt: Stadion Publishing Company, 1994.

Kreighbaum, Ellen and Barthels, Katharine M. Biomechanics - *A Qualitative Approach For Studying Human Movement*, Fourth edition. Boston, Allyn and Bacon. 1996.

Lee, Bruce. *Tao Of Jeet Kune Do*, Santa Clarita, California: Ohara Publications, Incorporated. 1975.

Logan, Gene A. and McKinney, Wayne C. *Kinesiology.* Wm. C. Brown Company Publishers. 1970.

Mackler, Lynn Snyder. *Scientific Rationale and Physiological Basis for the Use of Closed Kinetic Chain Exercise in Lower Extremity." Journal of Sports Rehabilitation*, Volume Five, # 5, February 1996.

McMahon, Thomas A. *Muscles, Reflexes, and Locomotion*, Princeton, New Jersey: Princeton University Press. 1984.

McArdle, William D. Katch, Frank I. And Katch, Victor L. (2001) Fifth Edition. Exercise *Physiology – Energy, Nutrition and Human Performance*, Baltimore, MD. Williams & Wilkins.

Olbrecht, Jan. *The Science of Winning – Planning, Periodizing and Optimizing Swim Training.* Swim Shop, Luton, England. 2000.

O'Shea, Patrick. (2000) *Quantum Strength Fitness II*, Corvallis, OR: Patrick's Books.

Palmtier, Randal A. An, Kai-Nan, Scott, Steven G. and Chao, Edmond Y.S. "Kinetic Chain Exercise in Knee Rehabilitation." *Sports Medicine*, Volume 11 #6 pp. 402-413, 1991.

Perrin, David H. *Anterior Cruciate Ligament Injury in the Female Athlete,* Journal of Athletic Training, Volume 34, #2, April-June 1999.

Radcliffe, James C. and Faentinos, Robert C. (1999) *High-Powered Plyometrics*, Champaign, IL: Human Kinetics Publishing Company.

Schmidt, Richard A. *Motor Control And Learning - A Behavioral Emphasis*, Second Edition. Champaign, Illinois: Human Kinetics Books, Inc. 1988.

Simpson, Kathy J. Ciaponni, Terri, and Wang, He. "*Biomechanics of Landing*" in Garrett, William E. and Kirkendal, Donald T. Editors. *Exercise and Sport Science,* Lippencott Williams & Wilkins, Pliadelphia. 2000.

Starzynski, Tadeusz. And Sozanski, Henryk. (1999) *Explosive Power and Jumping Ability for all Sports,* Island Pond, VT: Stadion Publishing Company.

Steele, Julie R. "*Landing Without Injury: Fact Or Fiction?*" In ISBS XVII International Symposium on Biomechanics in Sports Applied Proceedings: Fundamental Skills. Ross Sanders, Editor. Edith Cowen University, Perth Western Australia. 1999.

Todd, Mabel E. *The Thinking Body*, Princeton Book Company Publishers. Highston, NJ. 1937.

Wilk, Kevin E. Zheng, Naiquan. Fleisig, Glenn S. Andrews, James R. and Clancy, William G. "Kinetic Chain Exercise: Implicatios for the Anterior Cruciate Ligament Patient." *Journal of Sport Rehabilitation*, Volume Six, #2, May 1997.

Whiting, William C. and Zernicke, Ronald F. *Biomechanics of Musculoskeletal Injury*, (1998) Champaign, IL: Human Kinetics Publishing Company.

Zatsiorsky, Vladimir M. *Science and Practice of Strength Training*, (1995) Champaign, IL: Human Kinetics Publishing Company.

Zhuk, V. And Martynenko, N. "An alternative To Strength And Power Development For Young Athletes" *Modern Athlete And Coach*, Vol. 29 #3. July 1991.